Global Women's Health

Edited by Zhengchao Wang

Published in London, United Kingdom

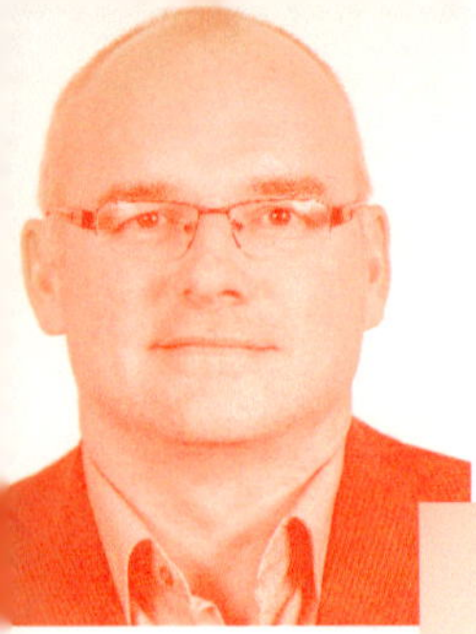
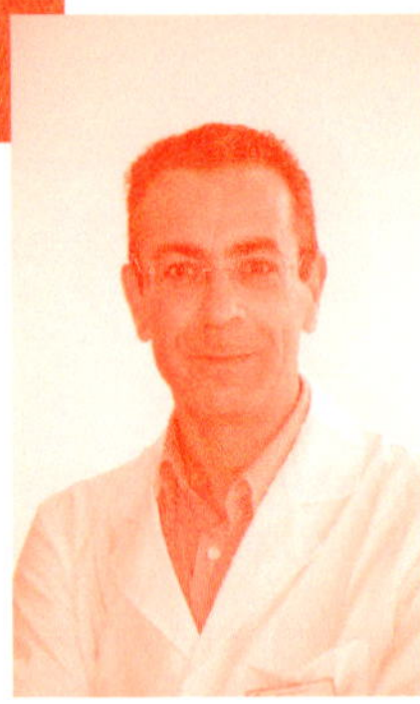
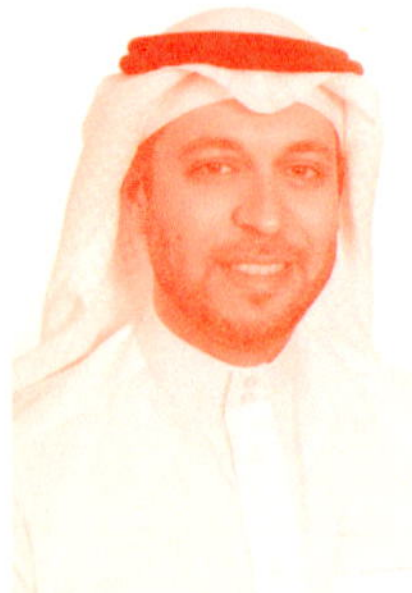
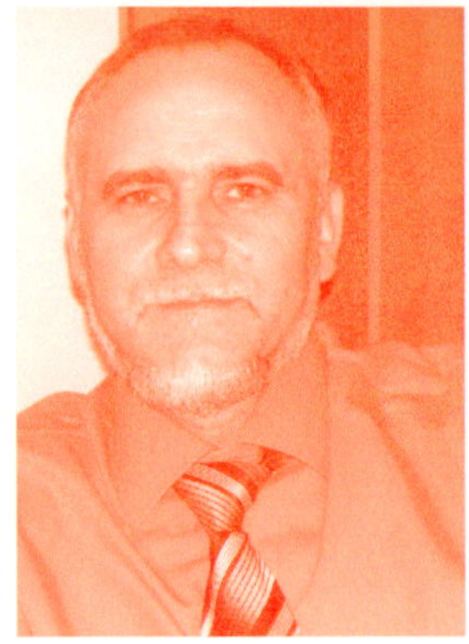
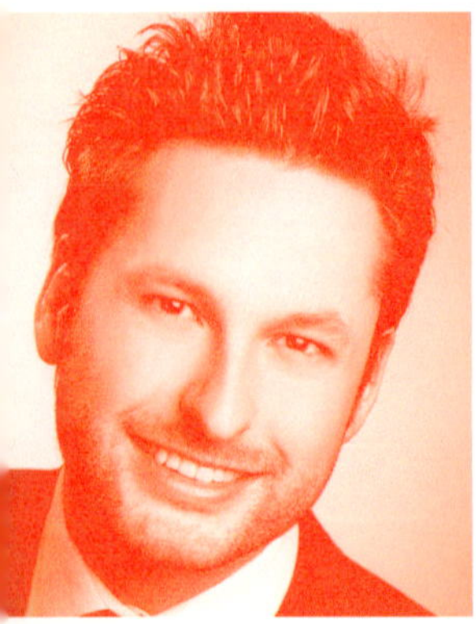
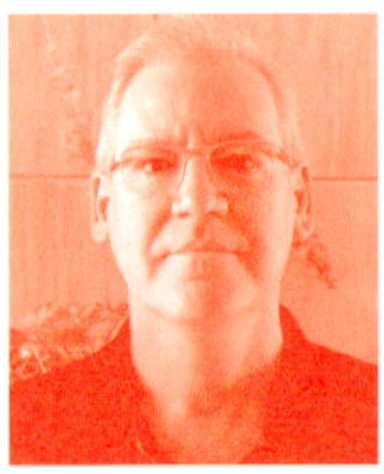
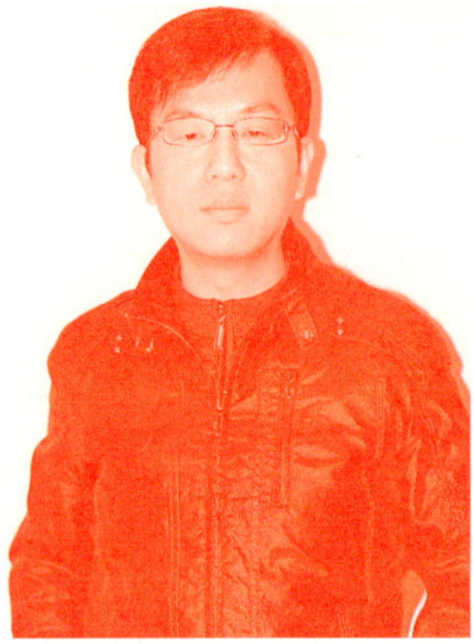

IntechOpen

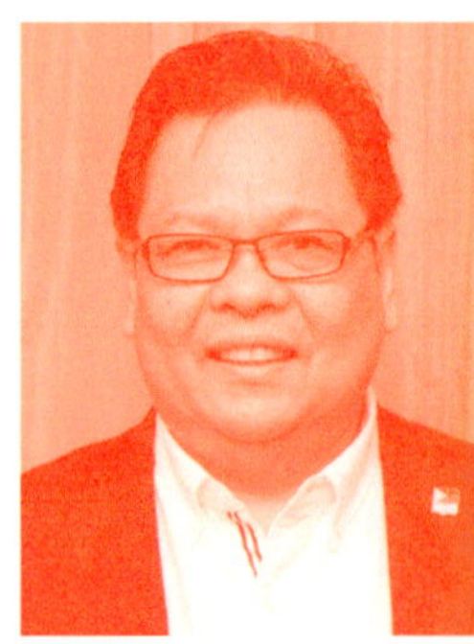
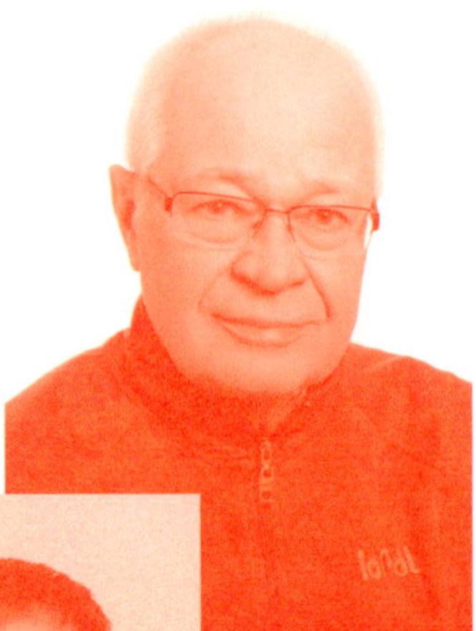
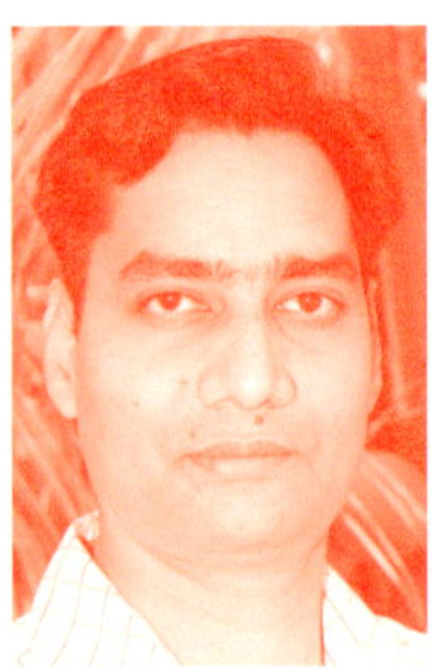
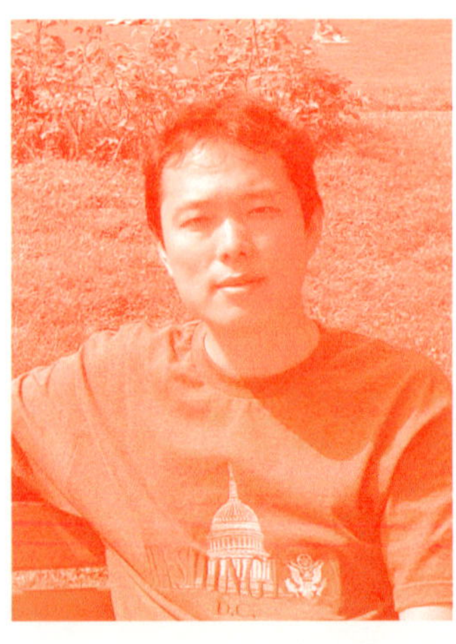
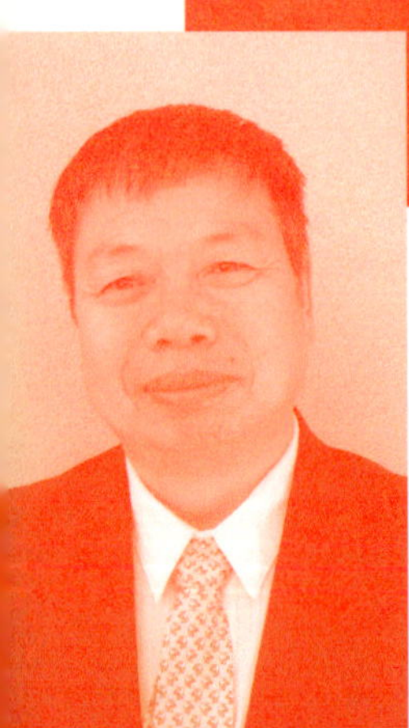
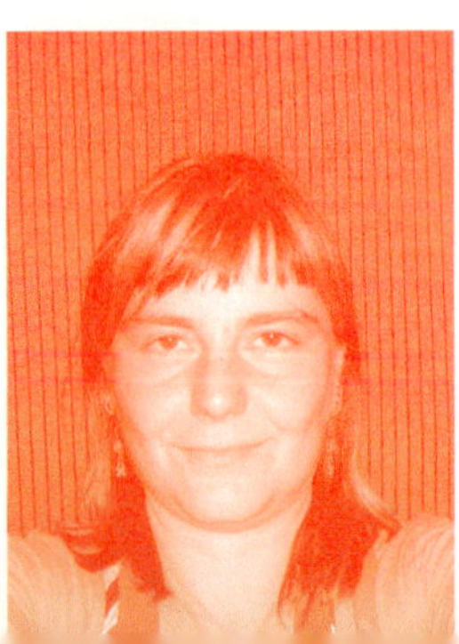

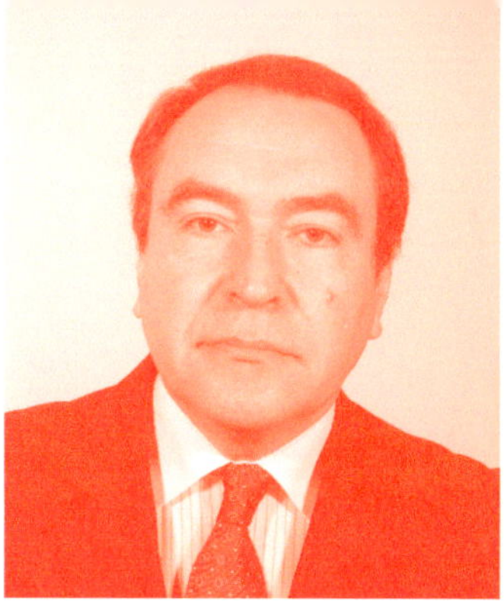
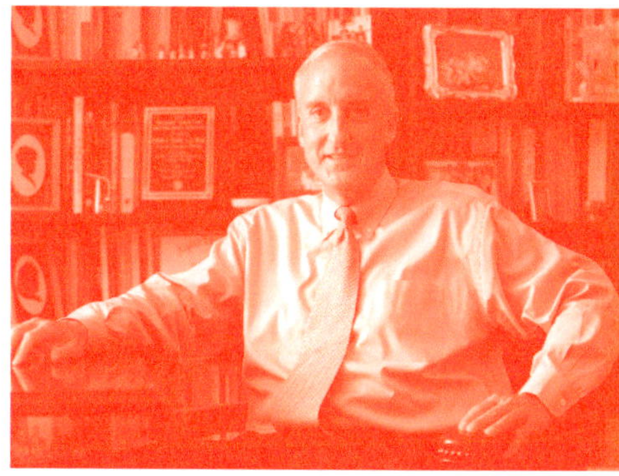
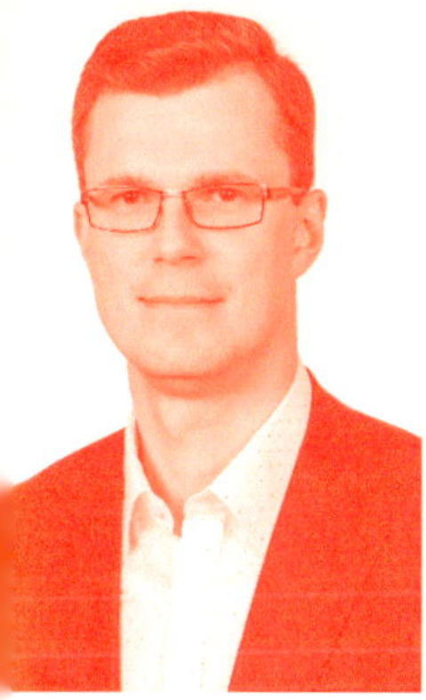
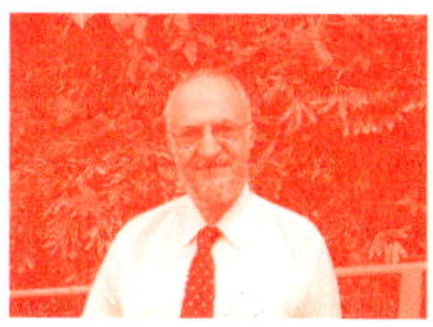
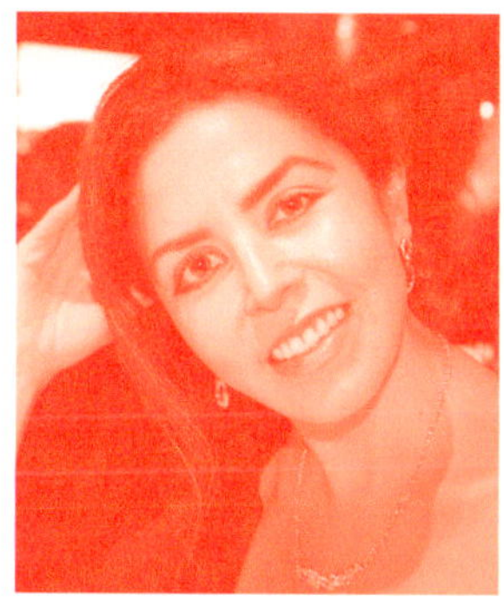

Supporting open minds since 2005

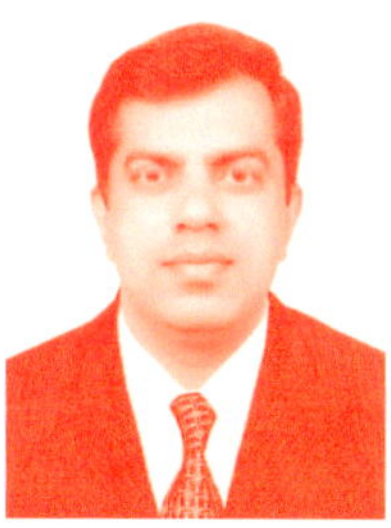
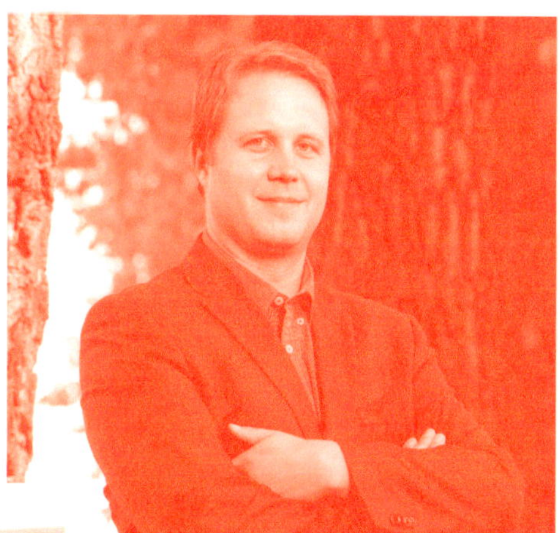
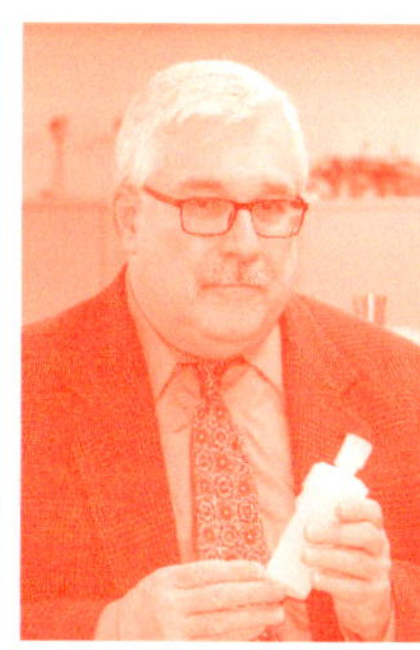
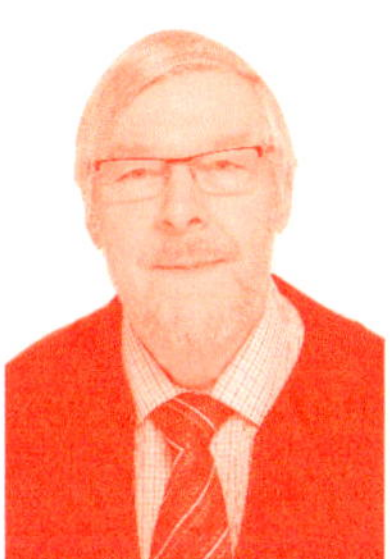
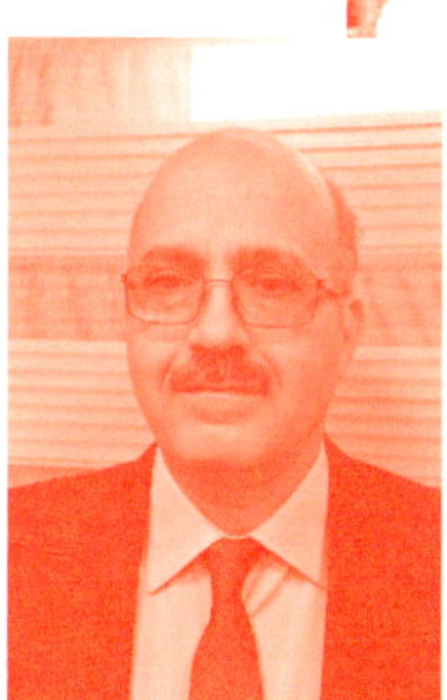
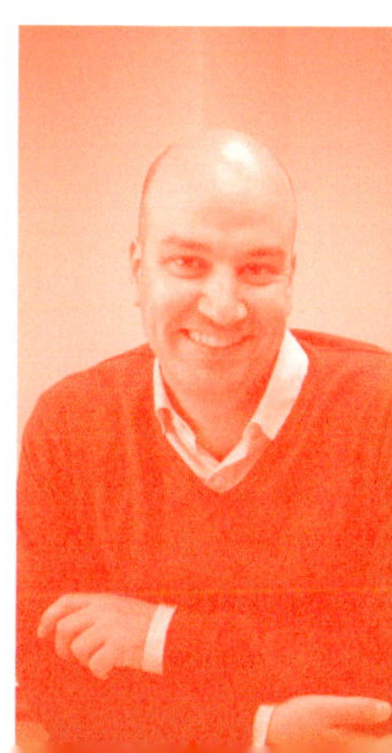
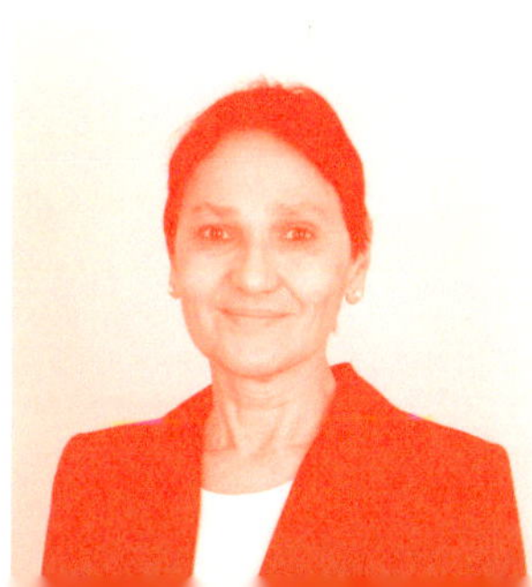

Global Women's Health
http://dx.doi.org/10.5772/intechopen.92947
Edited by Zhengchao Wang

Contributors
Amrit Pal Singh Rana, Manjit Kaur Rana, Congjian Shi, Hongqin Yang, Zhengchao Wang, Zhenghong Zhang, Nadeem Bilani, Zeina Nahleh, Leah Elson, Elizabeth Blessing Elimimian, Panagiotis Tsikouras, Riffat Mehboob, Fridoon Jawad Ahmad, Syed Amir Gilani, Sidra Khalid, Amber Hassan, Zainab Abdulameer Abdulrasol, Shazia Ali, Rabia Rashid, Pandurangan Ramaraj, Gayatri Devi Ramalingam, Saravana Kumar Sampath, Jothi Priya Amirtham, Anastasia Bothou, Aggeliki Gerede, Ifigenia Apostolou, Fotini Gaitatzi, Dorelia Deuteraiou, Anna Chalkidou, Xanthoula Anthoulaki, Spyridon Michalopoulos, Georgios Dragoutsos, Ioannis Tsirkas, Irini Babageorgaka, Theopi Nalbanti, Natalia Sachnova, Alexios Alexiou, Constantinos Nikolettos, Apostolos Lazarou, Stefanos Zervoudis, Panagiotis Peitsidis, Nikolaos Nikolettos, Hong Liang, Mahboob-Ul-Hussain

First published in London, United Kingdom, 2021 by IntechOpen
IntechOpen is the global imprint of INTECHOPEN LIMITED, registered in England and Wales, registration number: 11086078, 5 Princes Gate Court, London, SW7 2QJ, United Kingdom
Printed in Croatia

British Library Cataloguing-in-Publication Data
A catalogue record for this book is available from the British Library

Additional hard and PDF copies can be obtained from orders@intechopen.com

Global Women's Health
Edited by Zhengchao Wang
p. cm.
Print ISBN 978-1-83968-938-3
Online ISBN 978-1-83968-939-0
eBook (PDF) ISBN 978-1-83968-940-6

For EU product safety concerns:
IN TECH d.o.o., Prolaz Marije Krucifikse Kozulić 3, 51000 Rijeka, Croatia, info@intechopen.com or visit our website at intechopen.com.

Meet the editor

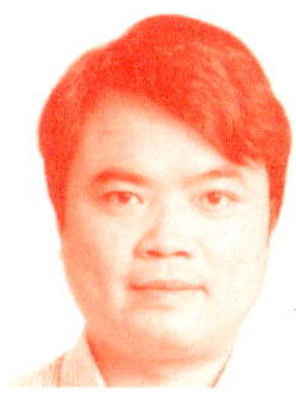

Dr. Zhengchao Wang is a full professor at the College of Life Sciences, Fujian Normal University, China. He is a Principal Investigator for the General Program for the National Natural Science Foundation of China and Program for New Century Excellent Talents in the University of Ministry of Education of China. He is also a team leader in the Fujian Provincial Key Laboratory for Developmental Biology and Neurosciences, Key Laboratory of Optoelectronic Science and Technology for Medicine of Ministry of Education. He obtained his Ph.D. in 2008 and has a long teaching and research career. He has published 172 scientific papers in English or Chinese, participated in approximately 32 grants, and published 12 books as the editor in his specialty and related diseases.

Contents

Preface

According to the United Nations, the global population in 2015 exceeded 7.3 billion, and the gender ratio gap between men and women is not large, which means that there are about 3.6 billion women in the world. Therefore, providing 3.6 billion women with high-quality healthcare services and quality is an important global concern. The global focus on women's health began in the 1970s. The United Nations designated 1975 as International Women's Year and 1976–1985 as the world's Decade for Women. In 1995, the Fourth World Conference on Women put forward the Beijing Declaration, with "equality, development and peace" as the main axis. Representatives of 189 countries jointly signed the Beijing Platform for Action, strongly advocated that countries should pay attention to women's issues, and began publishing "Current Situation and Future Trend of Global Women's Statistics." This publication addresses eight topics: population and family, health, education, work, rights and decision-making, violence against women, environment, and poverty. It describes the latest statistical data of women in the world and provides a brief analysis that can be used as a reference for countries to plan women's health policies and healthcare services. It is a world trend to attach importance to women's health. The United Nations Population Fund believes that the role of the government is very important if women are to have a bright future. The government is an important force to ensure women's right to health. The role of the government in promoting women's health should be reflected in the following aspects. The first is to support gender equality with legal policies, the second is to ensure the relationship between women workers and employers, and the third is to encourage research on gender-related issues. The 3.6 billion women in the world live in different countries, different social environments, different cultures, and different medical care systems, and each woman plays multiple roles and responsibilities, which highlights the diversity and complexity of women's health problems. Taking women as the main body, we should change the health inequality caused by the gender bias of social and cultural concepts, strengthen the integration strategy of cross fields and departments, and provide appropriate health plans and care for women taking into account ethnic groups, ages, causes of death, disease status and life events. This book provides a comprehensive overview of the current state of the art in global women's health, focusing on the most important evidence-based developments in this critically important area.

We sincerely thank Prof. Mehboob Riffat, Dr. Abdulrasol Zainab Abdulameer, Dr. Devi Gayatri, Prof. Tsikouras Panagiotis, Dr. Rana Amrit Pal Singh, Dr. Ramaraj Pandurangan, Dr. Congjian Shi, Dr. Bilani Nadeem, and Dr. Ali Shazia for their contributions.

Dr. Zhengchao Wang
College of Life Sciences,
Fujian Normal University,
Fuzhou, China

Section 1

Maternal Mortality and Life Quality

Chapter 1

Maternal Mortality Ratio in Low Income Developing Countries

Riffat Mehboob, Syed Amir Gilani, Sidra Khalid, Amber Hassan and Ahmad Alwazzan

Abstract

Maternal mortality (MM) is a matter of serious concern in low income developing countries (LDCs). A great reduction has been observed regarding the maternal deaths globally after huge efforts since 1990 todate. However, the situation continues to be either stagnant or worsening in developing countries, suggesting that the efforts to cope with this issue are either insufficient or not properly implemented. We need to first diagnose the problem areas that are a great hurdle in the road to success towards the reduction of MM. Postpartum hemorrhage and preeclampsia are one of the most common causes of MM. Malnutrition, neurological dysfunction and cancer are among the non-obstetric causes. Trained medical and paramedical staff can be of great help in this regard by increasing awareness among masses at grass root level. Target set by Millennium Development goal has minimized the MM by 44%. But it has not met the target set by Millenium Development Goals 5 and a lot of measures need to be taken in this regard. Majority of the MDs are preventable and can be avoided by adopting appropriate frameworks, linked data sets, surveillance, birth attendants training, preparation for births, etc. Delay in decision to get healthcare, access to healthcare center and receiving these facilities are the main factors in MM.

Keywords: maternal mortality, Pakistan, millenium development goals, sustainable development goals, antenatal care

1. Introduction

Severe Maternal Outcomes (SMO) comprises of Maternal Near Miss (MNM) or Maternal Death (MD) [1]. MD is considered as the most tragic event and can be preventable if the mother is given proper medical aid and facilities. It is considered as an indicator about the quality of medical services of a country [2]. WHO defines MD as: "the death of women during pregnancy or within 42 days after termination of pregnancy irrespective to the cause of death" [3]. Maternal Mortality Rate (MMR) is defined as the number of MDs divided by the number of live births during a particular time period [2]. A country's MMR indicates the development, health and medical status [4]. Maternal mortality (MM) is divided into direct and indirect deaths: direct death is caused by delivery and complication in 42 days of postpartum and indirect death are those MDs which are caused by any disease which is affected or enhanced by pregnancy's physiological effects. Accidental deaths in which pregnancy has no role is not considered as MD [2, 4, 5].

2. Trends in global mortality rates

Though MMR has decreased since 1990 to 2015 (estimated 303,000/100 million live births), it still remains a big challenge in many LDCs [6]. Some regions of the world have high MMR which is indicative of the poor health facilities and disparities in access. Low Income Developing countries (LDC) contribute to maximum of MMR (99%) [7, 8]. Sub-Saharan Africa has the highest MMR (14110/100 million live births) and South Asia (1428 million/100 million) is second in world ranking in 2015 while Common wealth Independent States including Armenia, Azerbaijan, Belarus, Georgia, Russia, Tajiskistan etc. has lowest (313/100 million live births) MMR. European Union also has second lowest MMR (307/100 million live births) (**Figure 1**). According to WHO report, the MMR in LDCs was 239 per 100 million live births as compared to 12 in developed countries (DC) in 2015. There are inequalities in these ratios between regions, countries, different socioeconomic strata, rural and urban populations [9].

Among South Asian countries, Afghanistan has the highest MMR (396/100 million live births) in 2015 while it was 1340/100 million live births in 1990, Pakistan is 7th in ranking in this region with 0.178 million/100 million live births in 2015 while it was 0.431 million/100 million live births in 1990. Srilanka has the lowest MMR (30/100 million live births) in 2015 while it was 75/100 million live births in 1990 (**Figure 2**) [10]. Siera Leone has an estimated MMR 1360/100 million live births which is not only highest in Sub-Saharan Afria but also in the world. Although it has dropped from 2630/100 million live births in 1990. Finland and Greece have the lowest MMR 3/100 live births globally and considered as best countries as far as maternal health is concerned (**Figure 3**) [10].

Globally the MMR has decreased from 385 in 1990 to 216 in 2015 showing an annual reduction of 2.3%. The yearly number decreased from 532 000 in 1990, to 303 000 in 2015. During 1990 to 2015, the annual reduction rate in Eastern Asia was 5·0% and in Caribbean was 1·8%. MMR of developed countries was 12/100 000 livebirths in 2015 and for Sub Saharan Africa was 546 respectively [8]. Globally large decline in different regions of the world has been observed that includes South-East Asia with 69% reduction and Western Pacific with 64% reduction. Least progress in MMR is observed in African with 44% decline and America with 49% decline [7, 8].

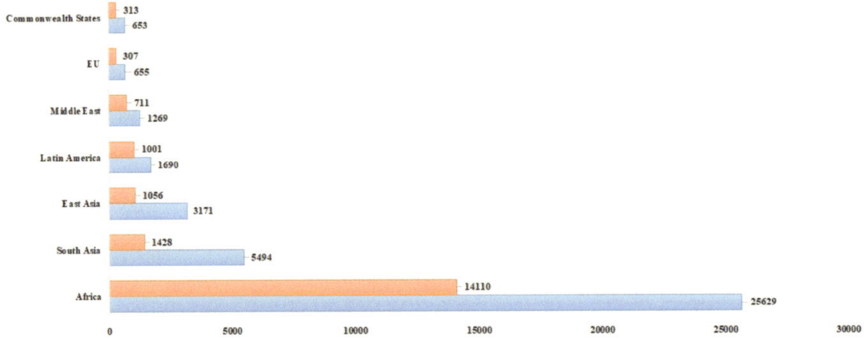

Figure 1.
Maternal mortality ratio (MD per 100 mllion live births) in 1990 and 2015 in different regions of world.

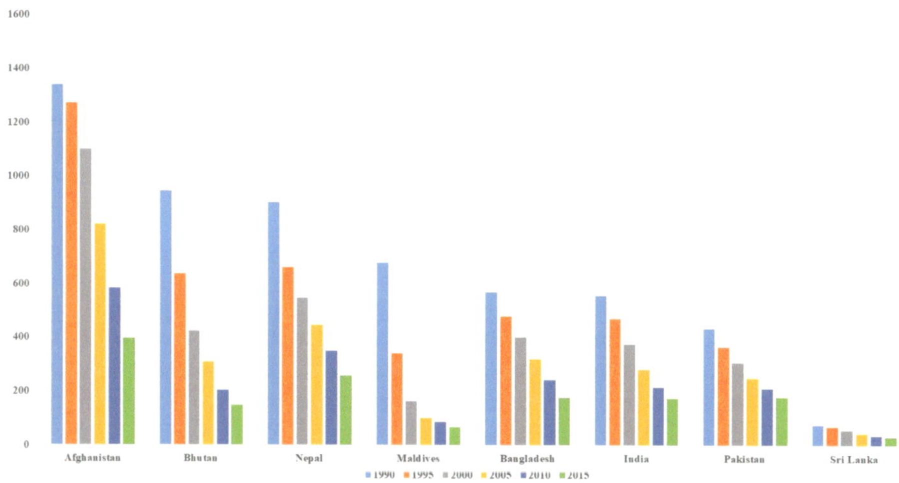

Figure 2.
Trends in MMR (1990–2015) in South Asia.

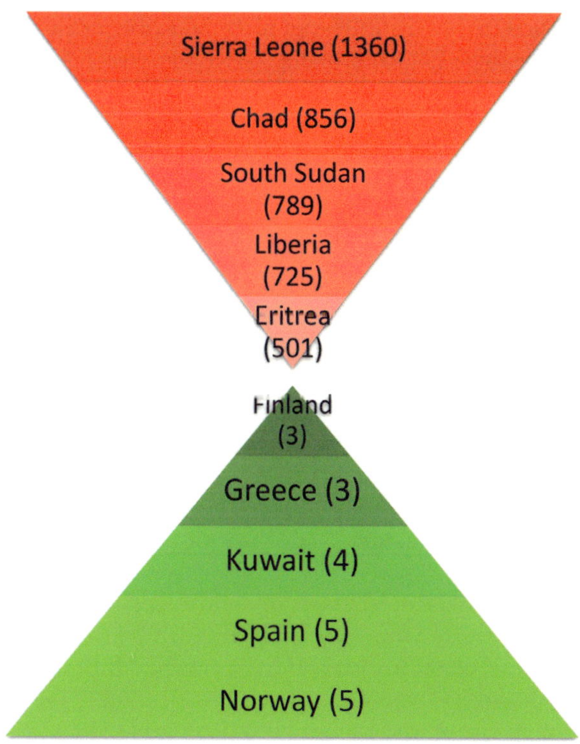

Figure 3.
Sand clock of five countries with highest (red) and lowest (green) MMR.

3. Millennium development goals and maternal mortality

Globally all organizations have focused on reducing MDs by initiating a number of programs since 1980's [5]. United Nations (UN) made 8 Millennium Development Goals (MDGs) in September 2000 in which one was about maternal mortality [11]. All the goals had to be achieved by the member countries by the end of 2015. MDG called for the reduction of 75% of maternal mortality by the end of 2015 and all countries and international agencies were directed to monitor the progress towards the completion of the goal (between 1990 to 2015) [8]. It means that the target would be achieved by maternal mortality decline of 5.5% per year during 25 years time period. However, MMR has decreased by 37% since 2000, even then 303 million women died across the world in 2015 [7].

4. Sustainable development goals-United Nations

International and national level political partnership and funding could improve education, socio-economic conditions, gender equality and environment. After end of era of MDGs a new agenda was announced in 2015 that consists of 17 SDGs [7]. According to SDGs the target is to decrease maternal deaths to <70 deaths per live births by 2030 and no country should increase its MMR to 140/100,000 live births [8, 12]. The United Nations (UN) secretary general Banki-Moon has started the global strategy for mothers, meonates, infants, children and Adolescent's health from 2016–2030 [13]. This Strategy will be a road map and tries to end all possible causes responsible for maternal mortality [8].

According to Goal 3.1 of Sustainable Development Goals (SDGs) of United Nations, MMR should be reduced to less than 70% per 100 million live births. Tremendous efforts have been made since 2000 and an impressive outcomes have been observed. Goal 3.7.1 focuses on women in their reproductive years, who had successfully adopted the modern family planning methods. Goal 3.7.2 discuss about the adolescent birth rate (10–19 years)/1000 women in that age group. MMR in sub-Saharan Africa has reduced by 35% since 2000. The adolescent birth rate in 2018 was 44/1,000 women (15–19 years) at global scale while 56 in the year 2000. Its rate is 101 in sub-Saharan Africa which is the highest of all. Target 3.7 addresses the availability and access to reproductive health, its awareness and implementation at national level, all over the world [14].

In 2010, 12% of global population spent approximately/10th of their budgets for health services as compated to 9.7% in 2000. An estimated $9.4 billion was donated from various donars as Official Development Assistance (ODA) in 2016 which is 41% more. All the data available so far indicates that 45% of the world and most of the LDCs (90%) have not even one physician per 1,000 population and approximately 60% have less than 3 nurses per 1,000 [14].

4.1 Maternal mortality in Pakistan

The status of MDs in Pakistan is very poor and Pakistan is recognized as a country with high MMR. It is estimated that approximately 30,000 women dies every year due to pregnancy-related complications [15]. Measuring MMR is also a big challenge due to poor system of record keeping and weak certification of the reason of causality [16]. The reduction rate of MMR from 1990–2015 was 3.5% with 431 MDs/100 million live births in 1990 to 178 deaths in 2015. 89% of deliveries occur at home that causes 80% of MDs. 80% delivery occurs by the traditional birth attendants (TBAs) and only 1 out of 20 pregnant women reaches hospital or dispensary emergency [17].

In a study conducted in a teaching hospital in Karachi indicated that unsafe abortions carried by untrained health care service providers was the main reason of MDs [18]. The most common among all reasons was hemorrhage and then eclampsia and sepsis [19]. Pre-eclampsia and eclampsia causes 10.4% and abortion cause 5.6% of MDs [16, 19]. The main reasons of MDs in another study from Khyber Pakhtunkhuwa (KPK) province of Pakistan were hemorrhage, sepsis, eclampsia, and hepatic encephalopathy. 40% of the overall cases were dealt by TDAs, 33% by lady health visitors, 17% received no care and 10% by doctors [20]. In a ten year study, from January 1995 to December

2004, conducted at Nishtar Hospital, Multan the major causative factors were hemorrhage, eclampsia, sepsis, anemia, and abortion. The study also concluded that increase in mother's age is linked to increased MDs [21]. Most of the studies concluded hemorrhage as the leading cause of death while sepsis or eclampsia was the second main cause. In indirect causes, anemia and hepatitis was the main cause of death [4].

Different studies have been conducted in the provinces and hospitals to identify main causes and prevention of MD [22]. In 2005, Jokhio *et al.* performed a cluster randomized controlled trial in seven regions (talukas) of a rural district Larkana, Sindh in Pakistan by training TBAs in three talukas known as intervention group and the remaining four talukas, TBAs were not trained (control group). The trained attendants were given sterilized delivery-kits for deliveries. 30% reduction in the intervention group was found as compared to the control group. This strategy can be applied to improve maternal health in LDCs [17].

Ali *et al.*, designed a study to gather information about the health care facilities and emergency obstetric care (EmOC) using unprocessed indicators, in Punjab and KPK. It was found that in Punjab only 16 and in KPK only 6 health care services provides these basic facilities. His study showed that basic Obstetric facilities are very poor in Pakistan and it is extremely necessary to increase access and upgradation of these services. Another important aspect is transportation as most of the hospitals in the study here lack functional ambulance to take patient immediately to a nearby hospital or health care facility. Only 5.7% of deliveries occured in government health care centers that provide EmOC. This shows that women who need basic treatment cannot access government hospitals but either go to private hospital or seek no care [17]. Midhat *et al.*, investigated the cause associated with MDs in 16 rural districts of Balochistan and KPK provinces of Pakistan. The study concluded that women under 19 and over 39 years, or those delivering for the first time and those with an earlier record of fetal loss were having a high risk of MD. Essential Obstetric Care (EOC) was linked to MD. Results showed that staffing of peripheral health facilities and the role of health care facility is also linked to MD, which needs to be improved [17].

4.2 Pakistan Demographic and Health Survey

A survey conducted by Pakistan Demographic and Health Survey (PDHS) reported the MMR as 276 during the year 2006–2007. Also, there are differences in MMR between different provinces such as MMR of Baluchistan was 785, Sindh 314, KPK 275 and Punjab was 227. Besides provincial differences, rural MMR (319) is double as compared to urban MMR (175). Pakistan progress towards completing Millenium Development Goals (MDG) was very inadequate due to lack of resources and failure to provide good health care services to pregnant women. According to PDHS, the set targets were not achieved by the end of 2015 [23]. The MMR in 1990 was 385 which dropped to 216 per 100 million live births in 2015. After the end of MDG of 2015, Sustainable Development Goals (SDGs) was stated that targets to reduce MMR by the end of 2030 is 70 maternal mortality per 100 million live births [7, 8]. Global MM has decreased between the years 1990–2015 to 44%. Although it did not meet the required target set by MDG5, still a lot of measures need to be done to meet the target [14].

4.3 The three delays model

This model was proposed by Thaddeus et al., in 1994. It proposes the contributing factors that lead to the maternal mortalities. According to this model, most of the factors: distance, cost and quality are preventable and can be avoided if the health care is provided intime without any delay. The three factors responsible for MDs are summarized in three delays model (**Figure 4**) [24].

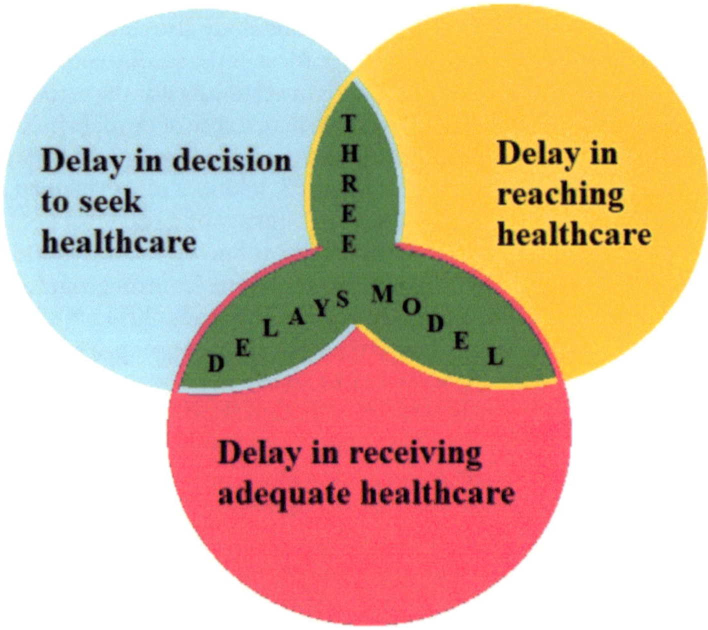

Figure 4.
The three delays model for maternal mortality.

4.4 Risk factors

Infrequent visits to Antenatal Care (ANC) units contribute substantially to the preventable MM in Sub-Saharan Africa. A home-based Community Health Worker (CHW) intervention in Tanzania significantly improved this situation in a locality with a higher level of facility based delivery. Policies should be devised and adopted to evaluate and design interventions to reduce the economic burden of ANC [25]. Inadequate training of midwives [26] and TBAs is a modifieable factor in reducing the MD [27]. In a retrospective study in Pakistan, those women who were administered by labour inducing medications by TBAs and lady health workers and susceptible for elongated duration of labour were more prone to uterine rupture and asphyxia while those with hemorrhage at the time of delivery (**Figure 5**) [26].

4.5 Eclampsia and hypertension

Approximately 42,000 MDs occured in the year 2015, as a result of pregnancy induced hypertension globally [28]. A study on 10 LDCs was conducted to evaluate the incidence of eclampsia and hypertension and its association to magnesion sulfate. 0.5% of all deliveries had eclampsia and 6.9% of them died. 0.95%/10,000 died from hypertension during pregnancy. These disparities in MDs across different LDCs is evident of inequality of availability and access to healthcare facilities for women with these complications in pregnancy (**Figure 5**) [28].

4.6 Postpartum hemorrhage (PPH)

Postpartum hemorrhage (PPH) was observed to have an association with MDs in Mozambique and Sub Saharan Africa [29, 30]. In 2015, the Mozambican Ministry of Health (MOH) launched a community-level misoprostol distribution program in chosen districts as a plan to decrease PPH. ExpandNet/World Health Organization

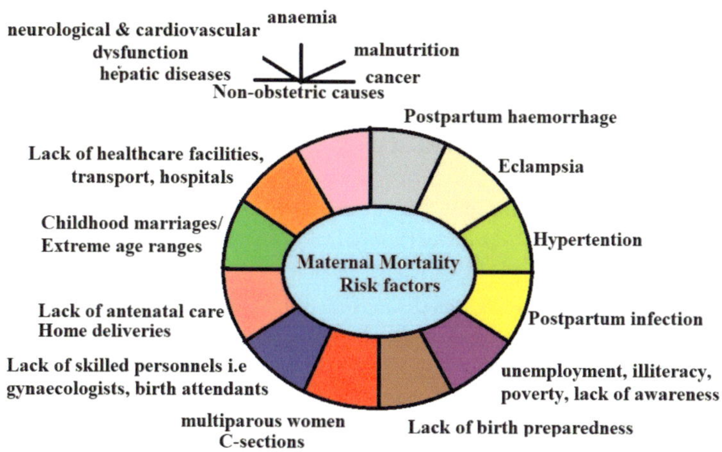

Figure 5.
Risk factors associated with maternal deaths.

(WHO) scale-up framework was used to evaluate the organization, evolution and the beneficial effects of misoprostol for the prevention of PPH. Interviews from health care staff and TBAs using the same framework in addition to national policies and 2017 guidelines from National Ministry of Maternal, newborn and childhealth workshop. The obstacles and accelerators associated with this program were highlighted in order to adapt this framework at national level [30]. The same causative factor was found to be linked to PPH and SMP in Nigeria. It occurred in 2.2% of the deliveries recorded in 42 tertiary care hospitals in Nigeria during one year period, among which 0.3% of women had an SMO [1]. Anemia may also lead to PPH (**Figure 5**) [31].

5. Non-obstetric causes of MDs

MNM was defined by WHO as an organ-system failure based on clinical criteria to assess the non-obstetric causes of SMO in a one year duration. It was observed that 9.4% (9401/100107) women admitted to the 42 tertiary hospitals in Nigeria for maternal complications had non-obstetric reasons. 4% (375/9401) of these complicated cases were MNM in 48% (183/375) and MD in 51.2% (192/375) [32]. Severe anemia contributed to 61.2% of MNM and 32.8% of MDs. Cancer contributed to the highest MI (91.7%), liver dysfunction (81.8%), HIV (80.4%), neurological (77.1%) and cardiovascular failures (75%). MDs were also associated with lack of awareness, lower and elderly ages. Consequently, it led to poorer pregnancy outcomes [32]. Similar findings were observed in another study in which the association of anemia with maternal and neonatal outcomes was investigated. Worldwide, 24.8% of population is anemic and pregnant women contributes the largest. It may lead to low birth weight, preterm delivery, low APGAR score etc. (**Figure 5**) [31].

6. Cesarean sections

MDs following cesarean sections are disproportionately high in LDCs. Timely access to the healthcare center is of utmost importance for a safe delivery. In a meta-analysis, 196 trials from 67 LDCs were analyzed. Women with C-section were at higher risk (7.6/1000 procedures). One-forth of all MDs in LDCs in 72 studies underwent C-section (**Figure 5**) [33].

7. Prevention of maternal mortality

MMR is difficult to measure. It is important to know the causes of MD and how it can be prevented. PDHS reports show that MD accounts for 20% of deaths of females of 15–49 years of age 0 [16, 23]. Most MDs can be prevented by providing care of skilled and trained personnel. All the causes discussed above can be prevented by giving proper diagnosis, management and understanding of childbirth problems [20]. Trained health professionals should handle labor complications. Severe bleeding can be stopped by an injection of oxytoxin. Also child birth should take place in hygienic environment. Pre-eclampsia can be prevented by giving drugs such as magnesium sulfate [19].

Main challenge is to provide proper EmOC 24/7. Staff training can increase confidence and skills. It is important to take steps for its implementation and upgrade basic plus comprehensive EmOC services [17].

8. Linked dataset for maternal outcomes

Linked dataset across any country or any population for assessing the maternal outcomes. In a recent study conducted in Australia, first national linked dataset was used for this purpose. Although, this data linkage had methodological and jurisdictional challenges, it is valuable source to enhance knowledge about maternal and neonatal outcomes from different settings (**Figure 6**) [34].

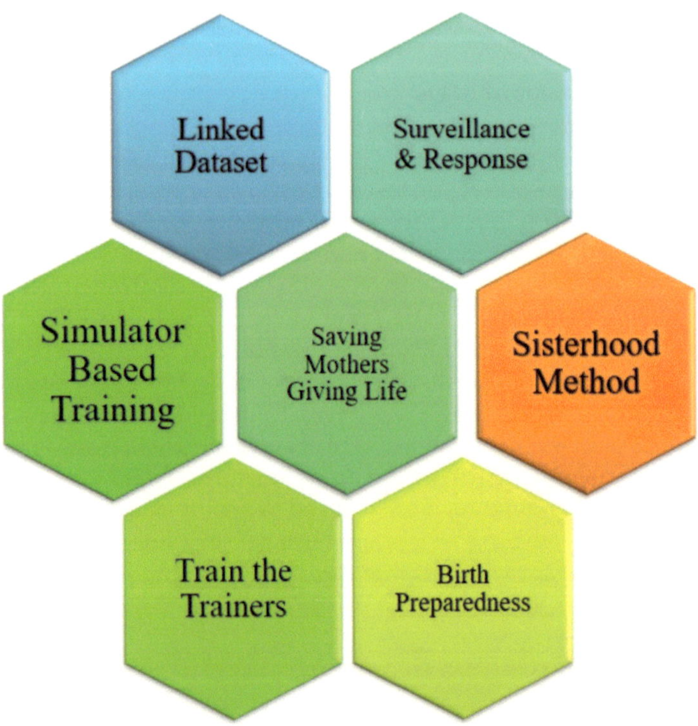

Figure 6.
Frameworks to prevent maternal deaths.

9. Sisterhood method of maternal mortality Surveillance

This method os surveillance is useful for estimation of MMRs in circumstances of limited resources, infrastructure and when mother is not available due to sad demise. Relatives, close family provide the information in such case. Based on National Total Fertility Rate (TFR) estimate of 4.88, Tajik Badakhshan had 141 MDs/100 million live births. Accurate TFRs are necessary for the actual and precise estimates of MD but certain variations are observed due to varied dempgraphics [35] (**Figure 6**).

10. Saving mothers giving life

Ending preventable MDs is still a worldwide problem that need to be address under the United Nations Sustainable Development Goal targets 3.1 and 3.2. [11]. Saving Mothers, Giving Life (SMGL) (**Figure 6**) was designed in 2011 within the Global Health Initiative as a public-private partnership between the U.S. government, Merck for Mothers, Every Mother Counts, the American College of Obstetricians and Gynecologists, the government of Norway, and Project C.U.R.E. SMGL's. The starting goal was to decrease the MDs in LDCs.

A pilot project was initiated under this approach (2012–2013) in 8 rural districts in Uganda and Zambia with high morbidity of MD. Later on it was expanded to 13 districts of Uganda and 18 of Zambia. The outcomes of this strategy after its implementation were marvelous. 35% decrease in MMR was observed in just one year, 44% in Uganda and 41% in Zambia during 5 years. Facilitated and assisted deliveries raised from 46–67% in Uganda, 62–90% in Zambia; C-sections increased from 5.3–9% in Uganda and 2.7–4.8% in Zambia; MDs reduced from 11.5–3-5% in Uganda and 10–5-2.8% in Zambia [36].

11. Simulator-based training

Simulator-based training may be beneficial and effective for the readiness and preparedness of TBAs and birth attendants in case of rare incidences or complications. It may save precious maternal and neonatal lives by improving the expertise and skills as well as preparing them for such events. Purpose is to establish the facilitators and obstacles in "low-dose, high-frequency" (LDHF) practice [29] (**Figure 6**).

12. Train the trainers Model

This model was adopted to conduct a course (2012–2015) in Cambodia to reduce the MDs. It was a sustainable model to create awareness and knowledge to improve the maternal outcomes. 3 hospitals and 42 health centers in Ethiopia were selected where the trainees collected the data and analyzed. A significantly high MMR was observed in cases of PPH, pre-eclampsia, complicated deliveries and C-sections. This ratio decreased from 64.7–40.8%/100 million deliveries in 2016 [37] (**Figure 6**).

13. Birth preparedness and complication readiness (BPCR)

This strategy helps the women to be aware of all possible maternal health care facilities during pregnancy and get ready for every circumstances including complications [6]. Ethiopia has the lowest antenatal care facilities due to low income and resources. Hence, it is creating awareness for BPCR through community services to reduce the MMR. In a study conducted in Ethiopia, secondary data from 215 women with a recent live birth in 10 health care centers was collected. Purpose of this survey was to get an insight regarding the birth readiness. Four out of six actions: identified a skilled health care provider, health center and transport, arranged the finances and clean delivery materials, prepared eatbles, were indicators of well preparedness of mothers. According to this criteria, two-third of the mothers were considered well prepared for delivery. Delivery in a health care center was practiced by well prepared mothers (57%). Antenatal birth preparedness counseling should be provided as a preventive measure to the mothers during the antenatal visits [38] (**Figure 6**).

14. Maternal Death Surveillance and Response (MDSR)

This system was proposed to provide knowledge for the prevention of MM. Evaluation of the MDSR was conducted in Hwange District, Zimbabwe, 2017.36 respondents were recruited from 11 health care centers, approximately 72% of them were women. Lack of knowledge and awareness of health care workers was found to be main reason for the late notification of MDs. MDSR system is reliable and useful but it is not very simple. Therefore, proper descriptions of the cases and guidelines for declaration of MDs should be taught and adopted by the heath care workers [39] (**Figure 6**).

15. Recommendations

According to the demand and suppy model to prevent MM, there are 4 needs of a balanced system: Health Promotion, Family planning, income generation and community advocacy. If these are provided, it will help in training of TBAs, upgraded equipents and provision of medicines, training of other health professionals by simulation based or other sessions and improvement in EmOC services. It may ultimately lead to the prevention or reduction in MMR [35] (**Figure 7**).

There is still a rise in MMR, despite of present stretegies to cope with this issue which is indicative of the insufficient obstetric, gynecological and neonatal care in LDCs [40]. Poor health and education in females is a matter of great concern in this regard. No monitoring body at government level is present to address these issues.

Strict control of labour/inducing drugs by the regulatory bodies is mandatory along with improved training of the healthcare workers [26]. Women with poorer access to the antenatal care facilities and skilled TBAs are at higher risk [41].

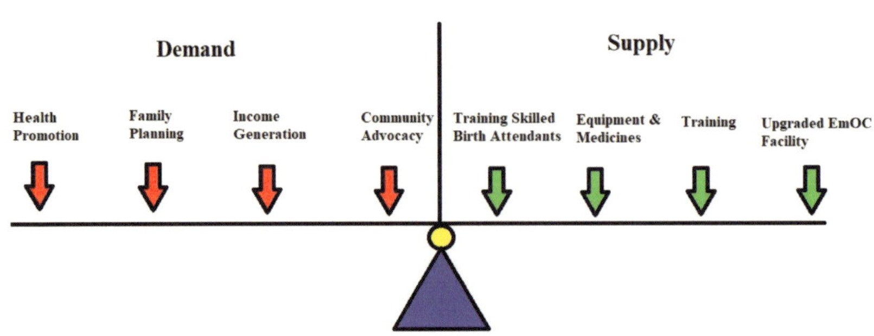

Figure 7.
Demand and supply model to prevent maternal mortality.

Efforts for the improvement of EmOC quality should be continued through proper skill-based training, incentives, latest equipment and sufficient drugs [42]. Education of females must be improved. Transportation should be improved for pregnant women as recommended in the UN-MDG-5 [43]. TBAs should be provided with financial benefits in recognition of referrals to community midwives [27]. Skilled TBAs assisted approximately 80% live births from 2012–2017 as compared to 62% from 2000–2005 [7]. Perspectives, concerns of different communities and the health care providers should be kept in mind before planning for any strategy, preventive measures, solutions and policies [44].

The rate of cesarean deliveries is alarmingly high in LDCs. Most of the patients go to private hospitals where cesarean deliveries are done just for commercial purposes [33]. Government should take strict measures to lower this negative trend. This undue practice is harmful not only for the health of mother but also for future pregnancies and their outcomes. Awareness classes should be compulsory for both parents in the case of first pregnancy as most of the observed mortalities are observed in primiparous mothers. Strategies should be devised for reduction of domestic violence. Laws should be enforced to minimize Intimate partner violence (IPV) during pregnancy. The Government should make policies and guidelines to improve maternal, child care and also for the antenatal care. Early marriages should be prohibited and laws should be enforced. Poor families should be given some support from government to bear the expenses of delivery, pre and post natal and maternal care. Better nutrition, health care facilities and education are needed to reverse these trends.

EmOC facilities should be improved at grass root scale of health care delivery to prevent avoidable MDs from PPH [1] and pre-eclampsis [45]. The adjustable parameters like maternal weight, diet, awareness and access to the health center should be monitored to improve the maternal and fetal situation and avoid MDs [46]. Proper implementation of these guidelines along with knowledge and training would guide the health professionals to diagnose the complications, manage them and help in reduction of MDs [6, 45, 47].

Research on maternal mortality in Pakistan is next to zero and there are no linked datasets, no coherent information. Hurdles are at both ends, Government (due to lack of resources, funds and priority) and people (they are not willing to investigate or provide information, poverty and lack of resources). These issues can be measured by a nation wide surveillance, coherent and linked datasets with all the information, and the models provided in this debate which are adopted by some other countries as well (simulator based training, train the trainers model, saving mothers giving life, birth preparedness, sisterhood method etc) may provide frameworks to the Government and healthcare policy makers to address and prevent this issue of serious concern to achieve the sustainable development goals.

Competing interests

Authors report no competing intestests or any conflict of interests.

Funding

No funding was received.

Ethical approval and consent to participate

N/A.

Consent for publication

Provided by all the authors.

Availability of data and material

It is a review and no data was used.

Authors contributions

All the authors have read and approved the final manuscript.

RM designed and planned the study. She supervised and mainly conceived the idea.

SAG facilitated the study, critically reviewed and helped in finalization of work.

SK also helped in write up and finalization.

AH helped in write up and compiling.

AA has critically reviewed and gave expert opinion.

Abbreviations

MM	Maternal Mortality
MNM	Maternal Near Miss
MMR	Maternal Mortality Ratio
MDGs	Millenium development goals
SDGs	Sustainable Development Goals
MD	Maternal Death
SMO	Severe Maternal Outcomes
LDC	Low Income Developing countries
DC	developed countries
ANC	Antenatal Care
ODA	Official Development Assistance
EmOC	emergency obstetric care
CHW	Community Health Worker
TBAs	Traditional Birth Attendants
PPH	Postpartum hemorrhage
MI	mortality index
CFR	case fatality rate
TFR	total fertility rate
LDHF	low-dose, high-frequency
MDSR	Maternal Death Surveillance and Response

Author details

Riffat Mehboob[1*], Syed Amir Gilani[2], Sidra Khalid[1], Amber Hassan[1] and Ahmad Alwazzan[3]

1 Research Unit, Faculty of Allied Health Sciences, The University of Lahore, Lahore, Pakistan

2 University Institute of Dietetics and Nutritional Sciences, Faculty of Allied Health Sciences, University of Lahore, Lahore, Pakistan

3 Division of Gynecology Oncology, Faculty of Medicine, King Abdulaziz University, Jeddah, Saudi Arabia

*Address all correspondence to: mehboob.riffat@gmail.com

References

[1] Sotunsa JO, Adeniyi AA, Imaralu JO, Fawole B, Adegbola O, Aimakhu CO, et al. Maternal near-miss and death among women with postpartum haemorrhage: a secondary analysis of the Nigeria Near-miss and Maternal Death Survey. BJOG: an international journal of obstetrics and gynaecology. 2019. Epub 2019/03/22.

[2] Wilmoth J, Mizoguchi N, Oestergaard M, Say L, Mathers C, Zureick-Brown S, et al. A new method for deriving global estimates of maternal mortality: Supplemental report. Available online from Statistics. Politics and Policy, http://www.degruyter.com/view/j/spp. 2012.

[3] Organization WH. International statistical classification of diseases and related health problems: World Health Organization; 2004.

[4] Jafarey S. Maternal mortality in Pakistan--compilation of available data. JPMA The Journal of the Pakistan Medical Association. 2002;52(12):539-544.

[5] Kassebaum NJ, Bertozzi-Villa A, Coggeshall MS, Shackelford KA, Steiner C, Heuton KR, et al. Global, regional, and national levels and causes of maternal mortality during 1990-2013: a systematic analysis for the Global Burden of Disease Study 2013. The Lancet. 2014;384(9947):980-1004.

[6] Azeze GA, Mokonnon TM, Kercho MW. Birth preparedness and complication readiness practice and influencing factors among women in Sodo town, Wolaita zone, Southern Ethiopia, 2018; community based cross-sectional study. Reproductive health. 2019;16(1):39. Epub 2019/03/31.

[7] Organization WH. Health in 2015: from MDGs, Millennium Development Goals to SDGs. Sustainable Development Goals Switzerland: World Health Organization Available: http://www.who.int/gho/publications/mdgs-sdgs/en/ [Accessed January 10 2016]. 2015.

[8] Alkema L, Chou D, Hogan D, Zhang S, Moller A-B, Gemmill A, et al. Global, regional, and national levels and trends in maternal mortality between 1990 and 2015, with scenario-based projections to 2030: a systematic analysis by the UN Maternal Mortality Estimation Inter-Agency Group. The Lancet. 2016;387(10017):462-474.

[9] Report WHO. https://www.who.int/news-room/fact-sheets/detail/maternal-mortality. Retrieved on 12 Feb 2018. 2018.

[10] World Health Organization U, United Nations Population Fund and The World Bank Trends in Maternal Mortality : 1990 to 2015, WHO, Geneva, 2015. https://datauniceforg/topic/maternal-health/maternal-mortality/. 2015.

[11] World Health Organization-Millenium Development Goals UN. https://www.who.int/topics/millennium_development_goals/about/en/. 2019.

[12] Organization WH. Strategies towards ending preventable maternal mortality (EPMM). 2015.

[13] WHO U. UNFPA, World Bank. Maternal mortality in 2005: estimates developed by WHO, UNICEF. UNFPA and the World Bank. Geneva: World Health Organization; 2007.

[14] World Health Organization-Sustainable Development Goals UN. https://sustainabledevelopment.un.org/sdg3. 2018.

[15] Jafarey S, editor. Maternal mortality in Pakistan: an overview

in maternal and perinatal health in Pakistan. Proceedings of an Asia and Oceania Federation of Obstetrics and Gynaecology (AOFOG) Workshop, Karachi; 1991.

[16] Jafarey SN, Rabbani A. Maternal mortality in Pakistan. National Committee on Maternal Health Newsletter. 2000.

[17] Gardosi J, Madurasinghe V, Williams M, Malik A, Francis A. Maternal and fetal risk factors for stillbirth: population based study. BMJ. 2013;346:f108. Epub 2013/01/26.

[18] Marufu TC, Ahankari A, Coleman T, Lewis S. Maternal smoking and the risk of still birth: systematic review and meta-analysis. BMC public health. 2015;15:239. Epub 2015/04/18.

[19] Altpeter F, Springer NM, Bartley LE, Blechl A, Brutnell TP, Citovsky V, et al. Advancing Crop Transformation in the Era of Genome Editing. The Plant cell. 2016. Epub 2016/06/21.

[20] Begum S, Aziz-un-Nisa BI. Analysis of maternal mortality in a tertiary care hospital to determine causes and preventable factors. J Ayub Med Coll Abbottabad. 2003;15(2):49-52.

[21] Lamont K, Scott NW, Jones GT, Bhattacharya S. Risk of recurrent stillbirth: systematic review and meta-analysis. BMJ. 2015;350:h3080. Epub 2015/06/26.

[22] Jafarey SN. Maternal mortality in Pakistan--compilation of available data. JPMA The Journal of the Pakistan Medical Association. 2002;52(12):539-544. Epub 2003/03/12.

[23] Newletter NCfMH. Maternal Mortality in Pakistan. https://wwwncmnhorgpk/wp-content/themes/ncmnh/images/ncmnh-newsletter-june-2000-newpdf. 2000.

[24] Thaddeus S, Maine D. Too far to walk: maternal mortality in context. Soc Sci Med. 1994;38(8):1091-1110. Epub 1994/04/01.

[25] Geldsetzer P, Mboggo E, Larson E, Lema IA, Magesa L, Machumi L, et al. Community health workers to improve uptake of maternal healthcare services: A cluster-randomized pragmatic trial in Dar es Salaam, Tanzania. PLoS medicine. 2019;16(3):e1002768. Epub 2019/03/30.

[26] Shah S, Van den Bergh R, Prinsloo JR, Rehman G, Bibi A, Shaeen N, et al. Unregulated usage of labour-inducing medication in a region of Pakistan with poor drug regulatory control: characteristics and risk patterns. International health. 2016;8(2):89-95.

[27] Shaikh BT, Khan S, Maab A, Amjad S. Emerging role of traditional birth attendants in mountainous terrain: a qualitative exploratory study from Chitral District, Pakistan. BMJ open. 2014;4(11):c006238. Epub 2014/11/28.

[28] Vousden N, Lawley E, Seed PT, Gidiri MF, Goudar S, Sandall J, et al. Incidence of eclampsia and related complications across 10 low- and middle-resource geographical regions: Secondary analysis of a cluster randomised controlled trial. PLoS medicine. 2019;16(3):e1002775. Epub 2019/03/30.

[29] Williams E BE, Holcombe S, Atukunda I, Namugerwa RI, Britt K, Evans C Practice so that the skill does not disappear": mixed methods evaluation of simulator-based learning for midwives in Uganda. BMC: Human Resources for Health. 2019;17(24).

[30] Hobday K, Hulme J, Prata N, Wate PZ, Belton S, Homer C. Scaling Up Misoprostol to Prevent Postpartum Hemorrhage at Home Births in Mozambique: A Case Study Applying

the ExpandNet/WHO Framework. Global health, science and practice. 2019;7(1):66-86. Epub 2019/03/31.

[31] Lumbanraja SN, Yaznil MR, Siregar DIS, Sakina A. The Correlation between Hemoglobin Concentration during Pregnancy with the Maternal and Neonatal Outcome. Open access Macedonian journal of medical sciences. 2019;7(4):594-598. Epub 2019/03/22.

[32] Adeniran AS, Ocheke AN, Nwachukwu D, Adewole N, Ageda B, Onile T, et al. Non-obstetric causes of severe maternal complications: a secondary analysis of the Nigeria Near-miss and Maternal Death Survey. BJOG : an international journal of obstetrics and gynaecology. 2019. Epub 2019/03/22.

[33] Sobhy S, Arroyo-Manzano D, Murugesu N, Karthikeyan G, Kumar V, Kaur I, et al. Maternal and perinatal mortality and complications associated with caesarean section in low-income and middle-income countries: a systematic review and meta-analysis. Lancet. 2019.

[34] Cheah SL, Scarf VL, Rossiter C, Thornton C, Homer CSE. Creating the first national linked dataset on perinatal and maternal outcomes in Australia: Methods and challenges. Journal of biomedical informatics. 2019:103152. Epub 2019/03/21.

[35] Liese KL, Pauls H, Robinson S, Patil C. Estimating Maternal Mortality in Remote Rural Regions: an Application of the Sisterhood Method in Tajikistan. Central Asian journal of global health. 2019;8(1):341. Epub 2019/03/19.

[36] Conlon CM, Serbanescu F, Marum L, Healey J, LaBrecque J, Hobson R, et al. Saving Mothers, Giving Life: It Takes a System to Save a Mother (Republication). Global health, science and practice. 2019;7(1):20-40. Epub 2019/03/31.

[37] Foo S, Tagore S, Mathur M, Poun K, Sam M, Tan KH, et al. A sustainable model to improve maternal health and promote early obstetric care in resource-poor regions. International journal of gynaecology and obstetrics: the official organ of the International Federation of Gynaecology and Obstetrics. 2019. Epub 2019/03/30.

[38] Rosado C, Callaghan-Koru JA, Estifanos AS, Sheferaw E, Shay T, De Graft-Johnson J, et al. Effect of Birth Preparedness on Institutional Delivery in Semiurban Ethiopia: A Cross-Sectional Study. Annals of global health. 2019;85(1). Epub 2019/03/30.

[39] Maphosa M, Juru TP, Masuka N, Mungati M, Gombe N, Nsubuga P, et al. Evaluation of the Maternal Death Surveillance and response system in Hwange District, Zimbabwe, 2017. BMC pregnancy and childbirth. 2019;19(1):103. Epub 2019/03/30.

[40] Pasha O, Saleem S, Ali S, Goudar SS, Garces A, Esamai F, et al. Maternal and newborn outcomes in Pakistan compared to other low and middle income countries in the Global Network's Maternal Newborn Health Registry: an active, community-based, pregnancy surveillance mechanism. Reproductive health. 2015;12 Suppl 2:S15. Epub 2015/06/13.

[41] McClure EM, Saleem S, Goudar SS, Moore JL, Garces A, Esamai F, et al. Stillbirth rates in low-middle income countries 2010-2013: a population-based, multi-country study from the Global Network. Reproductive health. 2015;12 Suppl 2:S7. Epub 2015/06/13.

[42] Utz B, Zafar S, Arshad N, Kana T, Gopalakrishnan S. Status of emergency obstetric care in four districts of Punjab, Pakistan - results of a baseline assessment. JPMA The Journal of the Pakistan Medical Association. 2015;65(5):480-485. Epub 2015/06/02.

[43] Budhwani H, Hearld KR, Harbison H. Individual and Area Level Factors Associated with Prenatal, Delivery, and Postnatal Care in Pakistan. Maternal and child health journal. 2015;19(10):2138-2146. Epub 2015/04/16.

[44] Hamid S, Malik AU, Richard F. Stillbirth--a neglected priority: understanding its social meaning in Pakistan. JPMA The Journal of the Pakistan Medical Association. 2014;64(3):331-3. Epub 2014/05/29.

[45] MacDonald EJ, Lepine S, Pledger M, Geller SE, Lawton B, Stone P. Pre-eclampsia causing severe maternal morbidity - A national retrospective review of preventability and opportunities for improved care. The Australian & New Zealand journal of obstetrics & gynaecology. 2019. Epub 2019/03/19.

[46] Wachamo TM, Bililign Yimer N, Bizuneh AD. Risk factors for low birth weight in hospitals of North Wello zone, Ethiopia: A case-control study. PloS one. 2019;14(3):e0213054. Epub 2019/03/21.

[47] Ntoimo LF, Okonofua FE, Ogu RN, Galadanci HS, Gana M, Okike ON, et al. Prevalence and risk factors for maternal mortality in referral hospitals in Nigeria: a multicenter study. International journal of women's health. 2018;10: 69-76. Epub 2018/02/15.

Chapter 2

Assessment of Primary Dysmenorrhea and Its Effect on the Quality of Life among Female Students at University of Babylon

Zainab Abdulameer Abdulrasol

Abstract

Primary dysmenorrhea (PD) is a painful menstrual flow in the absence of any pelvic pathology where pain is spasmodic in character and felt mostly in the lower abdominal area. PD considered as common problem in females at reproductive age, it's directly affects the quality of life (QoL). The main objective of this study is to find out the relationship between PD and QoL of among female students. Descriptive correlational study design carried out on (145) female students, purposive sampling, and their ages between (18–25) years, participants were selected from four faculties at the University of Babylon. Numeric rating pain scale (11-point scale) was used for assessing pain intensity, QoL has been assessed by the SF-36 health survey (SF-36). Data have been collected by using a structured interview as method of data collection and using questionnaire as study tool. Data were processed and analyzed by using SPSS version (25). The findings of the present study revealed that (62.1%) of respondents reported as severe primary dysmenorrhea. The greatest proportion of female students with fair QoL and (17.9%) with poor QoL. The study's finding finds out a negative significant correlation between PD intensity and overall QoL scale at $P \leq 0.05$ ($r = -0.642$, $P = 0.000$).

Keywords: primary dysmenorrhea, quality of life, female students, effect, assessment

1. Introduction

The transitional period of females from childhood to be sexually mature and become capable of production is termed as puberty. Throughout this transition several alterations will take place including hormonal, psychological, cognitive and physical changes besides to the evolution and sexual developments, these changes occur synchronously. The prime physiological change in girl life is the onset of menarche which is special event in females' life due to the first occurrence of menstruation [1].

Menstrual cycle is a natural phenomenon, it is a significant sign of females' health, and it is an important indicator of endocrine function. Yet, data on experience of menstrual cycle and its influence on the health conditions, quality of life (QoL) and social integration among females in developing countries are still insufficient [2].

Menstrual cycle is a periodical, cyclical and interim vaginal bleeding; begin with first occurrence of menstruation (menarche) until menopause. Moreover, its deemed as one of mammal's characteristics especially human, it is described as regular, repeated uterine bleeding depending on endometrial degeneration, that takes place each 21 to 35 days in normal regular menstrual period, within 2 till 6 days of blood flow and average of blood losses 20 to 60 mL, as general it persist up to 40 years [3, 4].

There are several structures of women's body that will cooperate with each other in order to initiate the menstrual blood flow, these structures are: hypothalamus, pituitary gland, ovaries, and uterus. All the four structures must play a part for the ovulation; menstruation commence when fertilization does not occur; menstruation (shedding of the endometrium) marks the beginning of the monthly cycle [5].

One of most common menstrual disorders is dysmenorrhea; which is an episode of uterine cramp in the lower abdominal segment, immediately before or during cycle, dysmenorrhea variance among women. There is lack in understanding the menstrual cycle disorders especially dysmenorrhea. Furthermore, lack of knowledge related to this condition among young girls because they receive scarce education on dysmenorrhea [6].

Dysmenorrhea is either primary which mean it is not related to pathological reasons or secondary related to pathological reasons. Primary dysmenorrhea (PD) occurs because of excessive amount of prostaglandin which is produced during the disintegration of pre-menstrual uterine endometrium. While, the pain is caused by a disorder in the women's reproductive organs, such as endometriosis, adenomyosis, uterine fibroid, or infections, called secondary dysmenorrhea. Pain severity may be measured by using scaled as "no pain, mild pain, moderate pain, severe pain and worst possible pain" [7].

Primary dysmenorrhea is frequent, yet is a challenging problem in Gynecology. Primary dysmenorrhea often, occurs in most if not all women; until this moment is still poorly understood and is seldom taken into consideration when assessing females' general health and life experiences [8].

PD clinical manifestation may include lower back pain, premenstrual irritability, nervousness, fatigue, depressed mood, headache, some of gastrointestinal symptoms such as; nausea, vomiting, bloated abdomen and difficulty in emptying the intestines with constipation or diarrhea, an urge to urinate frequently that can be noticeable in women with PD at least a part or for the duration of the menstrual period [9].

The clinical manifestations of primary dysmenorrhea have tremendous and negative effect on quality of life at least for several days from each calendar month. Primary dysmenorrhea is a complicated manifestation, that impacts on the quality of life and minimizes productiveness of females. An estimation that (50%) of teenagers and adult women or adolescent girls skipped schools or work at littlest once time because of feeling of discomfort and pain which is accompanied with menstrual cycle. This unrelieved acute pain of menstrual cycle can influence inversely on the pulmonary, cardiovascular, gastrointestinal, endocrine and immunity. In addition, the unrelieved chronic pain may inhibit the immunity, result in anger, fatigue, disability, and depression [10].

Primary dysmenorrhea as menstrual cycle disorder resulting in serious condition among women especially young females because its effect is not only about future fertility, it also affects their mental health and quality of life (QoL) [11].

Quality of Life is "defined as a subjective phenomenon based on individual perception, experiences, beliefs, and expectations. Nowadays, QoL has become an issue in many clinical studies" [12].

Wilson and Cleary (1995) suggest a model defining the process by which woman's physical health status, such as dysmenorrhea, effect on their quality of life (QoL). They put forward that both factors biological and psychological may result in physical and psychophysical manifestations, that probably later impact on functioning and quality of life [13].

Primary dysmenorrhea present features of acute and chronic pain; it is a recurring and regular onset of pain, in spite of its short time span. Yet, astonishingly few of females are known about what the impact of PD on the quality of life. There are extremely scant reports about emotional troubles in females who experiences periodical PD [14].

The most common cause for poorer quality of life is pain depending on precedent researches, QoL observed to be lesser in women with PD [15].

2. Research main body

2.1 Overview

Primary dysmenorrhea (painful periods) that are still little understood. PD is a clinical term used to describe pain that experienced during menstruation. PD is a significant clinical problem and results in considerable public health burden. Primary dysmenorrhea is not associated with any underlying pathological causes. The precise mechanisms responsible for the symptoms of primary dysmenorrhea are need to be elucidated [16].

The menstrual period is hormonally intermediated events which take place in four structures in the females' body. These females' biological structures are participating in the functioning of the menstrual period are: hypothalamus, pituitary gland, ovaries and uterine endometrium. For a menstrual period to initiate all 4 biological structures should collaborate; deactivate of any structure will results in an incomplete and ineffective period [17].

Primary dysmenorrhea increased rhythmic uterine contractions from vasoconstriction of small vessels of the uterine wall. This condition impacts a females' ability to achieve their daily activities for 2 or several days every month it is used to start within few years of the beginning of ovulatory cycles at menarche [18].

Degree of intensity include: mil, moderate, and severe; mild PD its agonize menstruation that rarely obstructs the normal activity and analgesics are rarely required, moderate pain is defined as aching menstrual cycle which impacts on daily activity and analgesic are necessary to give relief, in addition to severe pain which mean painful cycle which clearly obstructs daily activity and the pain is not completely relieved by analgesic [19].

Etiologies of PD are not exactly understood, but preponderance features may be clarified via an action of the uterine prostaglandin, generally. Prostaglandin (PGs) is ubiquitously diffused intra-cellular materials which is derived from the long chains poly-un-saturated fatty acid, like arachidonic acid, a usual ingredient of cells membrane phospholipids. Prostaglandins has existing to own a range of impacts on general range of biological and functional as pathological actions containing pain, inflammations, body temperature, also regulation of the sleep. PGs manufacturing and releasing is limited to an availability of free fatty acid predecessors for the arachidonic acid that regulated via cyclic adenosine phosphates. By the cyclical adenosine phosphates, PG manufacturing can be motivated via materials like adrenalin, a peptide hormone & the steroid hormone, besides the mechanical motivation and tissue injury [20].

Arachidonic acid is created from the phospholipids via a lysosomal enzyme phospholipase A2. The stability of the lysosomal activities regulated through several factors, one of these is the progesterone's level; the raised progesterone level tend to steady the activity of the lysosomes, on the other hand the dropping level tends to decrease the lysosome activity. Thus, the reduction in the progesterone's level will go along with the regression of corpus luteum in late luteal phase of menstrual period result in removal of this stabilizing impact on uterine endometrial lysosome, the releasing of phospholipase A2, menstrual period flow and hydrolysis of phospholipid from cell membrane to produce extra arachidonic acid [21].

Consequently, the continuing accessibility of arachidonic acid together with intracellular damage besides tissues' trauma through menstrual period, favoritism manufacturing of PGs. All the females have raised level of PGs during a luteal phase of period as comparison with the follicular phase of ovulatory periods. Though, as a comparison among females with eumenorrheic and females with primary dysmenorrhea, detected that the females with PD have upper level of PG, as measured in a luteal phase of endometrial biopsy [16].

The circulation of PGs (PGF2a & PGE2) is recorded higher level in females with primary dysmenorrhea as comparison with asymptomatic females throughout menstrual period, and this PG's level are uppermost in first forty-eight hours of menstrual period, when signs & symptoms topmost. Additionally, the severity of menstrual period's pain and accompanied features of primary dysmenorrhea are directly related to the amount of PGs that is released [22].

Moreover, when exogenous PGs is clinically administered lead to uterine contraction and produces identical systemic features which recurrently associated with primary dysmenorrhea, containing gastrointestinal symptoms; that means the PGs are causing painful uterine contraction and accompanied systemic clinical manifestations which is associated with primary dysmenorrhea [23].

On the basis that the endometrium is exposed to a luteal phase's progesterone its crucial to increase the production of uterine's PGs, primary dysmenorrhea supposed to happen just in the ovulatory menstrual period; while many studies has been challenged in terms of a basal body's temperature that utilized in order to differentiate between the ovulatory and anovulatory menstrual periods. There is no difference in the severity of menstrual periods symptoms, as well as pain, between the ovulatory and anovulatory menstrual periods among females with PD [24].

P.D. is a significant clinical problem and results in considerable public health burden. In 2007, an International Associations for the Study of Pain calculated roughly that those in every menstrual cycle, about 10% _15% of females with primary dysmenorrhea were incapable for working about 1–3 days. For example in the United States (U.S.), there is lost approximately (140) million of working hours because of PD every year. In Japan, it was predicted that monetary lost because of PD computed as $4.2 billion dollar every year. In India it has been detected that about 42% self-medicated and approximately 35% consumed unfitting drug and they used mefenamic acid as a NSAID in order to decrease the pain of PD [25].

Pain is considered as one of the major contributors for poor QoL. PD is a periodic pain state, in which females suffering from acute events of agonizing cramping during the menstrual periods. There is inadequate literatures on an associations among socio-demographical characteristics and menstrual cycle elements with severity of PD and the experiences of the female's students with PD to increase the understanding of phenomenon and the effects on the life of this group of sufferers [26].

Investigation of quality of life domains in females with primary dysmenorrhea manifestations has received very little attention. From menarche and throughout the pubertal years there are significant rise in depressive features and anxiety and smoking activities; it is critical to study that association of these problems with menstrual period disorders especially primary dysmenorrhea. The existence of both emotional and behavioral troubles can aggravate PD symptoms; it has been detected when evaluating the causes PD [27].

2.2 Methodology

2.2.1 Design of the Study

A descriptive correlational study design was carried out in order to assess the severity of primary dysmenorrhea, and its effect on quality of life among female students whose ages are between (18 to 25) years old, at the University of Babylon in the province of Babylon, from the period 1st September 2018 to 14th August 2019.

2.2.2 Administrative arrangements

Formal administrative agreements were acquired for conducting the current study before data collection. The Ethical Committee of the college of nursing approved the protocol for this study. Consent was attained from the University of Babylon from the colleges that involved as study's sitting which include; faculty of basic education, faculty of human education, college of engineering and college of science. Written consent was attained from the subjects undergone the study, any participant will have the right to retreat from the study at any time.

2.2.3 Setting of the study

The current study has been carried out in Babylon governorate at University of Babylon which consists of (21) colleges, (4) colleges were selected randomly to accomplish the study and then select department from each college as 10% randomly.

2.2.4 Study sample

A non-probability (purposive) sample; 30% of target population was selected of female students, were consisted of (145) participants. The selection included participants who have mild, moderate and sever intensity of primary dysmenorrhea. It is selected from (4) faculties.

2.2.5 The study instrument

Through the extensive review of relevant literatures and previous studies, a questionnaire constructed for the purpose of the study. It is composed of seven parts. The first one is demographic data, second part is Numeric Pain Rating Scale (NPRS), the third part is dietary habits, the fourth part is family history, the fifth part is pain reliever history, sixth part is menstrual history, and last one is SF-36 Health Survey of quality of life.

2.2.6 Method of data collection

After taking an approval from the institutional ethical committee, the data was collected. The participation of study subjects was on voluntarily basis, written consent obtained from female students who willing to participate. Data attained by utilization of the study tool (questionnaire) and face-to-face interview, structured interview as method of data collection. The investigator was available on the site during distribution of questionnaire, to explain for them the objectives behind the study and to avoid any form of misunderstanding and to facilitate accurate response by the subjects.

Data collection started from 9th of January 2019 to 13th of March 2019. Close end questions used in the questionnaire. Time was consumed for each interview approximately (15_20) minutes.

2.2.7 Methods of data analysis

The data of the present study was analyzed by the Statistical package of social science (SPSS) version (25). The tests which were used in this study were derived from both: descriptive and inferential statistic, which includes: frequencies, percentage, mean of scores, standard deviation, Chi-square and Pearson product–moment correlation; all of these tests were used in order to achieving the objectives of study.

2.3 Result

Table 1 reveals that a (61.1%) of the sample were within the age group (18–21) years old, the highest percentage represented (42.1%) of the female students are in second grade. According to the occupational status majority of participants (92.4%) were not working. The largest proportion of them sample were unmarried represented (89%). The table shows that (57.2%) were satisfied with their socio-economic condition; with respect to the sample address it has been found that (84.8%) of them live in the urban. Majority of them (95.9%) living with their families. Finally, (64.1%) of study sample were recorded a BMI (18.5 < BMI < 25).

As shown in **Table 2**, the highest percentage represented (62.1%) of the sample experience severe pain.

This table shows that the greatest proportion was tea consumers constituted (63.4%) and chocolate (62.1%), then (41.4%) cola, and coffee was (22.1%).

Table 4 demonstrate that the highest percentage was sister history of PD (56%), and (34.6%) belong to mothers history of PD while, (32%) belong to others such as aunts.

Table 5 shows that highest percentage of the sample constitutes (61.4%) used pharmacological relievers for primary dysmenorrhea during their menstrual period.

The table shows that highest percentage represented (61%) of the sample their age of menarche were between (13–15) years old; (52%) their duration of menstrual cycle between (3–5) days. Moreover, a (62.1%) of sample were with regular interval of menstrual cycle.

This table displays the mean of the subscales of quality of life which shows that most of sample with fair level of assessment related to the QoL domains.

The table has clarified that the majority (83.4%) of female students with fair QoL. While (9.0%) were with poor QoL.

In this table Pearson correlation coefficient was used in order to illustrate that there is a negative significant correlation between intensity of P.D. and QoL among female students at $P \leq 0.05$ ($r = -0.642$, $P. = 0.000$). The outcome of statistical test demonstrates that there is significant correlation between the average scores of study subjects with P.D. and overall QoL scale.

Variables	Groups	F	%
Age	18–21	89	61.4
	22–25	56	38.6
	Mean = 21.01	S.D. ± 1.557	
College's grade	First grade	23	15.9
	Second grade	61	42.1
	Third grade	14	9.7
	Fourth grade	47	32.4
Occupation	Working	11	7.6
	Not working	134	92.4
Marital status	Married	16	11.0
	Un married	129	89.0
Socioeconomic status	Satisfied	83	57.2
	Satisfied to some extent	54	37.2
	Not Satisfied	8	5.5
Address	Urban	123	84.8
	Rural	22	15.2
Residency	Living with family	139	95.9
	Dormitory	4	2.8
	Live with others	2	1.4
Body Mass Index	Below weight (BMI < 18.5)	6	4.1
	Normal weight (18.5 < BMI < 25)	93	64.1
	Over weight (BMI > 25)	46	31.7

f = frequency, % = percentage, SD = standard deviation.

Table 1.
Distribution of female students by their demographical characteristics (N = 145).

Dysmenorrhea intensity	F	%
Mild	18	12.4%
Moderate	37	25.5%
Severe	90	62.1%
Total	145	100%

f = frequency, % = percentage.

Table 2.
Numeric pain rating scale for assessing the intensity of primary dysmenorrhea in the female students (N = 145).

This table revealed that there was significant association between P.D. intensity and marital status. While, there were a non-significant associations with whole demographical data except marital status at $P \leq 0.05$.

This table revealed that there were significant and highly significant associations between P.D. intensity and overall SF-36 scale of quality of life at $p \leq 0.05$.

2.4 Discussion

Many studies and literatures emphasize that the sociodemographic characteristics are relate to most of the nursing subjects because nursing as a science deals with human being, people life, and health issues in different age groups and situations, the present study deals with the primary dysmenorrhea and its effect on QoL of female students; result show in **Table 1**, that high percent of sample undergone the study within age group (18–21) this may due to criteria of selection of the current study's sample, and the lawful age of students in colleges and universities; this result consistent with A cross-sectional study by Chia et al. [28].

Table 1 displayed that the highest percentage of them were female students in second grade, this might be due to the availability of the sample without interference from the researcher; while, the findings of cross-sectional study [29] to determine the prevalence and associated factors of primary dysmenorrhea and its impact to the students' daily activities, showed that the highest percent was first grade. Related the occupational status majority of respondents were not working, most of the students in this age group found to be busy with study requirements and they cannot enroll in any job specially the morning study's students.

In regard to the place of residency it has been found that the majority of female students that are living in urban as it displayed in **Table 1** and that finding matches with a cross-sectional study by Tawfeek [30], her result shown that most of sample from urban; while, findings of other study [30] carried on (900) girls from (8) schools; showed that (469) were of rural residence while (431) were urban ones.

In respect to the residential status the present study result reveals that almost all the female students were living with their families as illustrated in **Table 1** and that contrary to Habibi's [31] showed that the highest value belong to dormitory living.

The current study results revealed that majority of the sample were unmarried, that congruent with a descriptive study findings [32].

The findings of the present study in **Table 1** showed that more than fifty percent were satisfied with their socio-economic condition, which form the highest value, on the other hand, a cross-sectional study [33] exhibited that half of sample stated as satisfied to some extent; this variance may belong to the contentment that widely spreading in Iraqi community and that did not indicated in necessary they are with good socio-economic status but it give them sense of satisfying.

In the light of this study and regarding the BMI a high percentage of respondents were showed normal weight as clarified in **Table 1**, this finding is in line with study [34] confirmed that the majority had BMI within the standard range.

The findings in **Table 2** demonstrated the outcome of Numeric Pain Rating Scale for assessing pain severity; which shows the highest proportion reported sever pain then followed by moderate, and finally mild. It's well known that even with mild level of pain the quality of life of girls may be affected. The study's finding is not consistent to another study [11] that found only (17.7%) of their participants experience severe PD during their period.

In most cases of primary dysmenorrhea the girls may turn to some habits as well as some of those habits may have an influence on their condition. This study deals with them as variables. The results related to dietary habits as showed in **Table 3** which displayed that the highest percentage of sample were tea consumers; while non-of them was reported as smoker, this result as culture is true where most of our people are consuming tea most of their day time. This result seem to be close to findings of the study conducted by Faramarzi and Salmalian [35] in Iran on (360) medical science female students, they verified that most of their students drank tea.

The present study was revealed that all the participants had one or more than one family member or relative experience this pain as demonstrated in **Table 4**,

Dietary Habits	F	%
Cola	60	41.4%
Coffee	32	22.1%
Tea	92	63.4%
Chocolate	90	62.1%

f = frequency, % = percentage.

Table 3.
Dietary habits among female students with primary dysmenorrhea (N = 145).

Family History of PD	F	%
Mother history of PD	45	34.6%
Sister History of PD	73	56.2%
Others	42	32.3%

f = frequency, % = percentage.

Table 4.
Distribution of sample related to their family history of primary dysmenorrhea.

usually and in most conditions and cases like what this study concern with this type of variable is crucial because of the genetic factors. The current result disagree with a study [36] which indicate that most of their sample had no family history regarding to primary dysmenorrhea.

In regard to the pain relievers used by girls during PD, the results confirmed that more than half of them were using pharmacological substances during their period to reduce the cramps and pain discomforts as soon as possible as declared in **Table 5**, a study conducted [37] stated that more than half of their sample using pharmacological substances to relieved their pain.

The onset of menstruation is a part of maturation process, after retrieved articles documenting the menstrual history related to PD, studies revealed that the history of first period vary according to the country and the climate as well as the geographical area. It has been appeared from the current study that Mean and SD of menarche's age for females was (13 ± 1), usual menstrual duration (per days) was (5 ± 1) and more than half of the respondents were with regular menstrual period as illustrate in **Table 6**; a study [14] showed that Mean and SD of the age of menarche was (13 ± 2) and Mean & SD for menstrual period duration was (5 ± 1) these finding similar to current study's findings.

When assess the QoL among female students who experience PD **Table 7**, result revealed that majority of the females with fair QoL assessment, while only few stated good QoL as showed in **Table 8**. A study [9] proved that highest percentage was with poor QoL, with negative impact on the QoL, mainly as related to

Pain reliever	F	%
Pharmacological	89	61.4%
Non pharmacological	54	37.2%
Hormonal therapy	2	1.4%

f = frequency, % = percentage.

Table 5.
Pain relievers history used with primary dysmenorrhea (N = 145).

Variables	Groups	F	%
Age of Menarche	10–12 years	51	35%
	13–15 years	88	61%
	Above 15 years	6	4%
Mean = 13.15		SD ± 1.249	
Duration of Cycle	3–5 Day	76	52.5%
	6–8 Day	69	47.5%
Mean = 5.57		SD ± 1.279	
Type of Cycle	Regular	90	62.1%
	Irregular	55	37.9%

f = frequency, % = percentage.

Table 6.
Menstrual characteristics for female students with primary dysmenorrhea.

Quality Rank	QoL's rating	F	%
Poor QoL	1–1.66	13	9.0
Fair QoL	1.67–2.33	121	83.4
Good QoL	2.34–3	11	7.6
Total		145	100%

Table 7.
Assessment of overall quality of life scale of female students with primary dysmenorrhea (N = 145).

university attendance and performance and social relationships. Tanmahasamut and Chawengsettakul [38] agreed with current study's findings, they confirm PD in students has high prevalence and it has result in poor quality of life.

The current study illustrated a negative significant correlation between the average scores of study subjects with P.D. and overall QoL scale at $P \leq 0.05$ (r = −0.642, p = 0.000), in other words when severity of P.D. pain level increase the quality of life decrease as introduced in **Table 9**. A descriptive study [39] reported that the reduction in QoL was clearly linked to the presence of primary dysmenorrhea.

The present study demonstrated that there is no significant association between socio-demographical features and the intensity of P.D except with marital status as displayed in **Table 10**; there are limited studies on an association of P.D intensity and socio-demographical characteristics.

Present study findings incompatible with a study [33] which accentuated in their results that the risk of primary dysmenorrhea increase in those who had lower incomes as well as in those with family history of P.D. Another study [40] similar to current study's findings revealed that there was no significant association between pain relievers use, dietary habits, and BMI of students with PD, except for coffee consumption at ($P < 0.001$); also no significant association between menstrual cycle characteristics and primary dysmenorrhea was revealed except for menstrual period bleeding duration and family history.

The current study showed in **Table 11** that there were mostly significant and highly significant associations between P.D. intensity and overall SF-36 scale of quality of life at $\boldsymbol{p \leq 0.05}$. Pain has negative impact on females' life, especially during menstrual period, because it's accompanied with hormonal alterations; that

NO.	Items	Never	Sometimes	Always	Mean	Ass.
General health domain:						
1.	In general, would you say your health is good?	27	108	10	2.12	Fair
2.	Compared to one year ago, you would say that your health in general is better now?	38	71	36	2.01	Fair
3.	I seem to get sick a little easier than other people	42	54	49	1.95	Fair
4.	I am as healthy as anybody I know	33	84	28	2.03	Fair
5.	I expect my health to get worse	21	79	45	1.83	Fair
6.	My health is excellent	35	85	25	2.07	Fair
	Domain mean = 2.0016		Assessment = Fair			
Limitation of activities domain:						
1.	Do you find difficulty while performing Vigorous activities, such as running, lifting heavy objects, participating in strenuous sports?	52	68	25	2.19	Fair
2.	Do you find difficulty while doing Moderate activities, such as moving a table, pushing a vacuum cleaner, bowling, or playing golf?	35	58	52	1.88	Fair
3.	Do you find difficulty when Lifting or carrying groceries?	25	59	61	1.75	Fair
4.	Do you find difficulty when Climbing several flights of stairs?	50	61	34	2.11	Fair
5.	Do you find difficulty when Climbing one flight of stairs?	80	45	20	2.41	Good
6.	Do you find difficulty when Bending, kneeling, or stooping?	80	46	19	2.42	Good
7	Do you find difficulty when Walking more than a mile?	37	63	45	1.94	Fair
8.	Do you find difficulty when Walking several blocks?	27	60	58	1.79	Fair
9.	Do you find difficulty when Walking one block?	43	45	57	1.90	Fair
10.	Do you find difficulties when Bathing or dressing yourself?	105	29	11	2.64	Good
	Domain mean = 2.1031		Assessment = Fair			
Physical health problems domain:						
1.	Cut down the amount of time you spent on work or other activities	23	94	28	1.97	Fair
2.	Accomplished less than you would like	32	83	30	2.01	Fair
3.	Were limited in the kind of work or other activities	35	54	26	2.06	Fair
4.	Had difficulty performing the work or other activities (for example, it took extra effort)	33	90	22	2.08	Fair
	Domain mean = 2.0293		Assessment = Fair			
Emotional health problems domain:						
1.	Cut down the amount of time you spent on work or other activities	38	87	20	2.12	Fair
2.	Accomplished less than you would like	31	94	20	2.08	Fair

NO.	Items	Never	Sometimes	Always	Mean	Ass.
3.	Didn't do work or other activities as carefully as usual	35	75	35	2.00	Fair
	Domain mean = 2.0665		Assessment = Fair			
Social activities domain:						
1.	Have you had emotional problems interfered with your normal social activities with family, friends, neighbors, or groups?	47	63	35	2.08	Fair
2.	During the menstrual cycle, most of the time your physical health or emotional problems interfered with your social activities (like visiting with friends, relatives, etc.)?	49	78	18	2.21	Fair
	Domain mean = 2.1483		Assessment = Fair			
Pain domain:						
1.	Have you had bodily pain during the menstrual cycle?	13	64	68	1.62	Poor
2.	During the menstrual cycle, have you had pain interfere with your normal work (including both work outside the home and housework)?	55	73	17	2.26	Fair
	Domain mean = 1.9403		Assessment = Fair			
Energy and emotion domain:						
1.	Did you feel full of pep?	26	87	32	1.96	Fair
2.	Have you been a very nervous person?	52	70	23	2.20	Fair
3.	Have you felt so down in the dumps that nothing could cheer you up?	43	75	27	2.11	Fair
4.	Have you felt calm and peaceful?	30	90	25	2.03	Fair
5.	Did you have a lot of energy?	24	82	39	1.90	Fair
6.	Have you felt downhearted and blue?	38	79	28	2.07	Fair
7.	Did you feel worn out?	43	79	23	2.14	Fair
8.	Have you been a happy person?	21	90	34	1.91	Fair
9.	Did you feel tired?	54	72	19	2.24	Fair
	Domain mean = 2.0613		Assessment = Fair			

Ass. = assessment, level of assessment: (1–1.66) as poor level, (1.67–2.33) as fair level and (2.34–3) as good level of QoL.

Table 8.
Distribution of female students according to their quality of life (SF-36) scale.

		Primary dysmenorrhea intensity
Quality of life	*r*	−.642-**
	Sig.	.000
	N	145

r = *(Pearson correlation), sig = (significant).*
*** Correlation is significant at the 0.01 level.*

Table 9.
Correlation between quality of life & primary dysmenorrhea.

Sociodemographic variable	Primary dysmenorrhea intensity			Chi-square test			
Age	**Mild**	**Moderate**	**Severe**	**X^2**	**D.F**	**P value**	**Sig.**
18–21	9	19	61	7.980	6	.240	NS.
22–25	9	18	27				
Marital status							
Married	5	3	8	5.885	2	.050	S
Single	13	34	82				
Socioeconomic status							
Satisfied	10	22	51	5.483	4	.241	NS.
Satisfied to some extent	8	15	31				
Not Satisfied	0	0	8				
Address							
Urban	16	35	72	4.603	2	.100	NS.
Rural	2	2	18				
Residency							
Living with family	17	35	87	1.386	4	.847	NS.
Hostel	1	1	2				
Live with others	0	1	1				
BMI							
Below weight (BMI < 18.5)	0	2	4	3.372	6	.761	NS.
Normal weight (18.5 < BMI < 25)	10	23	60				
Over weight (BMI > 25)	8	12	26				
Tea							
Yes	13	21	58	1.350	2	.509	NS.
No	5	16	32				
Chocolate							
Yes	12	26	52	1.923	2	.382	NS.
No	6	11	38				
Family history							
Yes	16	32	82	.618	2	.734	NS.
No	2	5	8				
Pain relievers history							
Pharmacological	10	21	58	2.566	4	.633	NS.
Non pharmacological	8	16	30				
Hormonal therapy	0	0	2				
Type of cycle							
Regular	13	24	53	1.298	2	.523	NS.
Irregular	5	13	37				

X^2 = Chi-square, D.F. = degree of freedom, P. value = probability, sig. = significance, S. = significant, H.S. = highly significant, N.S. = not significant.

Table 10.
Association of primary dysmenorrhea intensity with some variables.

Association of PD intensity with QoL							
General health domain	**Mild**	**Moderate**	**Severe**	**X^2**	**D.F**	**P value**	**Sig.**
Poor	7	5	20	10.018	4	.040	S
Fair	10	32	60				
Good	1	0	10				
Limitation of activities							
Poor	1	2	17	8.035	6	.236	NS.
Fair	9	17	45				
Good	8	18	28				
Physical health							
Poor	1	4	29	19.677	8	.012	H.S
Fair	11	21	50				
Good	6	12	11				
Emotional health							
Poor	3	11	39	11.991	8	.152	NS.
Fair	13	18	43				
Good	2	8	8				
Social activities							
Poor	1	7	51	40.822	8	.000	H.S
Fair	6	22	24				
Good	11	8	15				
Pain domain							
Poor	0	2	75	210.944	8	.000	H.S
Fair	0	34	15				
Good	18	1	0				
Energy and emotion							
Poor	2	9	19	5.016	6	.542	NS.
Fair	15	26	65				
Good	1	2	6				

X^2 = Chi-square, D.F. = degree of freedom, P. value = probability, sig. = significance, S. = significant, H.S. = highly significant, N.S. = not significant.

Table 11.
Association of primary dysmenorrhea intensity with quality of life (SF-36) scale.

basically cause some aliments to most of females. A study [12] supported this result and found that primary dysmenorrhea adversely affect the QoL.

3. Conclusions

According to the findings and discussion of the study's findings it can be concluded that higher percentage of the sample aged of (18–21) and living in urban region. Majority of these female students were unmarried, their socioeconomic status was satisfied. More than half of respondents were with severe primary dysmenorrhea. Majority the participants had positive family history of Primary dysmenorrhea. More than half of the study's sample appeared with regular period. Most of results showed that respondents using pharmacological agents as strategies of pain relief. The great majority domains of the quality of life showed fair assessment regarding primary dysmenorrhea. Present study shows that when primary dysmenorrhea intensity increases the quality of life will decrease. All the demographic data showed insignificant correlation with primary dysmenorrhea except the marital status. A significant to high significant association was found between primary dysmenorrhea intensity and quality of life.

Author details

Zainab Abdulameer Abdulrasol
University of Babylon, College of Nursing, Babylon, Iraq

*Address all correspondence to: saraaameer44a@gmail.com; nur.zainab.abdulameer@uobabylon.edu.iq

References

[1] Sutar, A., Paldhikar, S., Shikalgar, N., & Ghodey, S. (2016). "Effect of aerobic exercises on primary dysmenorrhoea in college students." IOSR Journal of Nursing and Health Science, 05(05), 20–24. https://doi.org/10.9790/1959-0505052024.

[2] Santina, T., Wehbe, N., and Ziade, F. (2012). Exploring dysmenorrhoea and menstrual experiences among Lebanese female adolescents. Eastern Mediterranean Health Journal, 18(8), 857–863.

[3] Silva, F., Mukai, L., Vitalle, M., & Medeiros, É. (2004). Prevalência de dismenorreia em pacientes avaliadas no centro de atendimento e apoio ao adoloscente da Universidade Federal de São Paulo. Rev. Paul. Pediatr, 22(2), 85–88.

[4] Brown, J., & Brown, S. (2010). Exercise for dysmenorrhoea. In J. Brown (Ed.), journal of Cochrane Database of Systematic Reviews. https://doi.org/10.1002/14651858.CD004142.pub2.

[5] Pillitteri, A. (2010). Maternal and Child health Nursing : Care of the Childbearing and Childrearing Family (6th ed.). philadelphia: Lippincott Williams & Wilkins.p.87-113.

[6] Harel, Z. (2006). Dysmenorrhea in adolescents and young adults: etiology and management. Journal of Pediatric and Adolescent Gynecology, 19(6), 363–371. https://doi.org/10.1016/j.jpag.2006.09.001

[7] Fraser, D. M., & Cooper, M. A. (2003). MA, Myles' Textbook for Midwives. London: Churchill Livington. p.149.

[8] Koninckx, P. R., Ussia, A., Adamyan, L., Keckstein, J., & Wattiez, A. (2017). Primary Dysmenorrhea. Journal of Obstetrics and Gynaecology Canada, 39 (7), 578–579. https://doi.org/10.1016/j.jogc.2017.03.093.

[9] Al-Jefout, M., Seham, A.-F., Jameel, H., Randa, A.-Q., Ola, A.-M., Oday, A.-M., & Luscombe, G. (2015). Dysmenorrhea: Prevalence and Impact on Quality of Life among Young Adult Jordanian Females. Journal of Pediatric and Adolescent Gynecology, 28(3), 173–185. https://doi.org/10.1016/j.jpag.2014.07.005.

[10] Smeltzer, S., Bare, B., Hinkle, J., and Cheever, K., (2008). Brunner & Suddarth s Textbook of Medical-Surgical Nursing. (11th ed.). Philadelphia, Lippincott Williams and Willkins. p.1168.

[11] Kazama, M., Maruyama, K., & Nakamura, K. (2015). Prevalence of Dysmenorrhea and Its Correlating Lifestyle Factors in Japanese Female Junior High School Students. The Tohoku Journal of Experimental Medicine, 236(2), 107–113. https://doi.org/10.1620/tjem.236.107.

[12] Joshi, T., Kural, M., Agrawal, D., Noor, N., & Patil, A. (2015). Primary dysmenorrhea and its effect on quality of life in young girls. International Journal of Medical Science and Public Health, 4(3), 381. https://doi.org/10.5455/ijmsph.2015.0711201472.

[13] Hardy-johnson, P., Graham, C., Creighton, S., & Liossi, C. (2014). The Impact of Dysmenorrhea on Young People's Health-Related Quality of Life. Journal of National Institute for Heaith Research, 1–25.

[14] Iacovides, S. (2013). The Impact of Primary Dysmenorrhoea on Pain Perception, Quality of Life, and Sleep in Young Healthy Women. University of the Witwatersrand, Johannesburg. https://doi.org/10.1017/CBO9781107415324.004.

[15] Rahmati, M., & Far, M. H. (2017). Comparing the Life Quality of Female Students with and without Primary Dysmenorrhea in Zahedan University of Medical Sciences in 2016. World Family Medicine Journal/Middle East Journal of Family Medicine, 15(10), 265–271. https://doi.org/10.5742/MEWFM.2017.93172.

[16] Jabbour, N., Kelly, W., Fraser, M., & Critchley, O. (2006). Endocrine regulation of menstruation. Journal of Endocrine Reviews, 27(1), 17–46. https://doi.org/10.1210/er.2004-0021.

[17] Ward, S., and Shelton, M. (2009). Maternal-Child Nursing CarMaternal-child nursing care: optimizing outcomes for mothers, children, and families. Philadelphia.p.138-140.

[18] Taylor, H. S., Adamson, G. D., Diamond, M. P., Goldstein, S. R., Horne, A. W., Missmer, S. A., Taylor, R. N. (2018). An evidence-based approach to assessing surgical versus clinical diagnosis of symptomatic endometriosis. International Journal of Gynecology & Obstetrics, 142(2), 131–142.

[19] Al-Kindi, R., & Al-Bulushi, A. (2011). Prevalence and Impact of Dysmenorrhoea among Omani High School Students. Sultan Qaboos University Medical Journal, 11(4), 485–491. Retrieved from https://www.ncbi.nlm.nih.gov/pubmed/22087397.

[20] Funk, C. D. (2001). Prostaglandins and leukotrienes: advances in eicosanoid biology. Journal of Science, 294(5548), 1871–1875.

[21] Fortier, M. A., Krishnaswamy, K., Danyod, G., Boucher-Kovalik, S., & Chapdalaine, P. (2008). A postgenomic integrated view of prostaglandins in reproduction: implications for other body systems. Journal of Physiol Pharmacol, 59(Suppl 1), 65–89.

[22] Dawood, M. Y. (2006). Primary dysmenorrhea: advances in pathogenesis and management. Journal of Obstetrics & Gynecology, 108(2), 428–441.

[23] Parent, J., & Fortier, M. A. (2005). Expression and contribution of three different isoforms of prostaglandin E synthase in the bovine endometrium. Journal of Biology of Reproduction, 73 (1), 36–44.

[24] Espín, L. L., Carrillo, E. V., González, F. J., Ordoñana, J. R. M., & Gomez-Amor, J. (2010). Incidence of anovulatory menstrual cycles among dysmenorrheic and non-non-dysmenorrheic [corrected] women: effects on symptomatology and mood. Journal of Psicothema, 22(4), 654–658.

[25] Gibson, S. J. (2007). IASP global year against pain in older persons: highlighting the current status and future perspectives in geriatric pain. Journal of Expert Review of Neurotherapeutics, 7(6), 627–635.

[26] Saeed, A. A. (2018). Associated Clinical Manifestations and Self - management Approaches of Primary Dysmenorrhea among Adolescent Students in Erbil City, Iraq. 150–154. https://doi.org/10.4103/MJBL.MJBL.

[27] Lorah, D., Sonya, N., Bin, H., Stephanie, P., Jennifer, H., Paula, B., and Susman, J. (2009). Menstrual Symptoms in Adolescent Girls: Association with Smoking, Depressive Symptoms and Anxiety. 44(3), 237–243. https://doi.org/10.1038/mp.2011.182.doi.

[28] Chia, C. F., Lai, J. H., Cheung, P. K., Kwong, L. T., Lau, F. P. M., Leung, K. H., Ngu, S. F. (2013). Dysmenorrhoea among Hong Kong university students: prevalence, impact, and management. Hong Kong Medical Journal = Xianggang Yi Xue Za Zhi, *19*(3), 222–228. https://doi.org/10.12809/hkmj133807.

[29] Tawfeek, R. S. (2008). Impact of dysmenorrheal among sample of female students in Tikrit University at 2008. Tikrit Medical Journal, 14(2), 127–130.

[30] Aziem, A., Ali, A., Rayis, D. A., Mamoun, M., & Adam, I. (2011). Age at menarche and menstrual cycle pattern among schoolgirls in Kassala in eastern Sudan. Journal of Public Health and Epidemiology, 3(3), 111–114. Retrieved from http://www.academicjournals.org/jphe.

[31] Habibi, N., Huang, M. S., Gan, W. Y., Zulida, R., & Safavi, S. M. (2015). Prevalence of Primary Dysmenorrhea and Factors Associated with Its Intensity Among Undergraduate Students: A Cross-Sectional Study. Journal of Pain Management Nursing, 16(6), 855–861. https://doi.org/10.1016/j.pmn.2015.07.001.

[32] Emmanuel, A., Achema, G., Gimba, S., Mafuyai, M., Afoi, B., & Ifere, I. (2013). Dysmenorrhoea: Pain relief strategies among a cohort of undergraduates in Nigeria. International Journal of Medicine and Biomedical Research, 2(2), 142–146. https://doi.org/10.14194/ijmbr.227.

[33] Assefa, N., Demissie, A., & Hailemeskel, S. (2016). Primary dysmenorrhea magnitude, associated risk factors, and its effect on academic performance: evidence from female university students in Ethiopia. International Journal of Women's Health, Volume 8, 489–496. https://doi.org/10.2147/IJWH.S112768.

[34] Shaik, S. A., Hashim, R. T., Alsukait, S. F., Abdulkader, G. M., AlSudairy, H. F., AlShaman, L. M., Fouda Neel, M. A. (2015). Assessment of age at menarche and its relation with body mass index in school girls of Riyadh, Saudi Arabia. Asian Journal of Medical Sciences, *7*(2), 5–12. https://doi.org/10.3126/ajms.v7i2.13439.

[35] Faramarzi, M., & Salmalian, H. (2014). Association of Psychologic and Nonpsychologic Factors with Primary Dysmenorrhea. Iranian Red Crescent Medical Journal, 16(8). https://doi.org/10.5812/ircmj.16307.

[36] Charu, S., Amita, R., Sujoy, R., & Thomas, G. A. (2012). "Menstrual characteristics" and "Prevalence and Effect of Dysmenorrhea" on Quality of Life of medical students "Menstrual characteristics" and "prevalence and effects of dysmenorrhea" on quality of life of medical students. International Journal of Collaborative Research on Internal Medicine & Public Health, 4 (4), 276. https://doi.org/ISSN1840-4529.

[37] Abu Helwa, H. A., Mitaeb, A. A., Al-Hamshri, S., & Sweileh, W. M. (2018). Prevalence of dysmenorrhea and predictors of its pain intensity among Palestinian female university students. Journal of BMC Women's Health, 18(1), 18. https://doi.org/10.1186/s12905-018-0516-1.

[38] Tanmahasamut, P., & Chawengsettakul, S. (2012). Dysmenorrhea in siriraj medical students; prevalence, quality of life, and knowledge of management. Journal of the Medical Association of Thailand, *95* (9), 1115–1121.

[39] Kannan, P., Chapple, C. M., Miller, D., Claydon, L. S., & Baxter, G. D. (2015). Menstrual pain and quality of life in women with primary dysmenorrhea: Rationale, design, and interventions of a randomized controlled trial of effects of a treadmill-based exercise intervention. Journal of Contemporary Clinical Trials, 42, 81–89. https://doi.org/10.1016/j.cct.2015.03.010.

[40] Unsal, A., Ayranci, U., Tozun, M., Arslan, G., & Calik, E. (2010). Prevalence of dysmenorrhea and its effect on quality of life among a group of female university students. Upsala Journal of Medical Sciences, *115*(2), 138–145. https://doi.org/10.3109/03009730903457218.

Section 2

Pregnancy and Preterm Labour

Chapter 3

Challenges Facing during Pregnancy and Measures to Overcome

Gayatri Devi Ramalingam, Saravana Kumar Sampath and Jothi Priya Amirtham

Abstract

Pregnancy is a time of transformation for both the mother and the baby, with significant physical and emotional changes. There are many discomforts that occur during pregnancy. Morning sickness, headache and backache, bladder and bowel changes, changes in hair and skin colour, indigestion and heartburn, leg cramps and swelling, vaginal thrush and discharge are the few common complications facing during pregnancy. As a result, the aim of this study was to describe the difficulties in obtaining health information and the measures to overcome the discomfort during pregnancy. Research articles for this review were searched by using the keywords "pregnancy", health issues", "measures to overcome", "challenges". There were studies that looked at the health problems that women face during pregnancy were included in this review article. Pregnancy issues such as gestational diabetes mellitus, hypertension, preeclampsia, caesarean birth, and postpartum weight retention are all more likely in overweight and obese women. More research into the link between nutritional advancements and the rising prevalence of GDM in the developing world is needed. Iron supplementation has been linked to glucose dysregulation and hypertension in mid-pregnancy; its effectiveness and potential risks should be carefully considered. As a result, legislators and health planners should remove barriers, promote self-care, and improve the quality of life for pregnant women, ultimately improving their health.

Keywords: Pregnancy, management, gestational diabetes, Preeclampsia, Anaemia

1. Introduction

Pregnancy is a time of transformation for both the mother and the baby, with significant physical and emotional changes. Even in uncomplicated pregnancies, these improvements can impact pregnant women's quality of life as well as maternal and child health. Women's wellbeing, as well as their current level of understanding and knowledge, would undoubtedly have a significant impact on society [1]. Pregnant women need health information to improve their self-care skills and increase their empowerment when following preventive health habits. The cardiovascular system undergoes various changes as a result of pregnancy. A normal, healthy pregnant woman's blood volume rises by nearly 50% over that of a non-pregnant woman. In addition, due to the vascular permeability associated with extreme preeclampsia, efforts to increase blood volume in these patients have been unsuccessful [1, 2]. Pregnancy (critical care scenario) is the reduction in venous return to the heart and decrease in cardiac output associated with the supine position. This effect is obviously more pronounced in the third trimester, when the uterus is largest. The so-called supine hypotensive syndrome.

When treating a critically ill pregnant woman, various hematologic changes must be taken into account. During pregnancy, the thrombocyte count remains largely constant, it leads to thrombocytosis. These improvements, when combined with a decrease in fibrinolysis, lead to the hypercoagulable state of pregnancy. Deep vein thrombosis and pulmonary embolism are five times more common during and immediately after pregnancy [3]. Both the residual volume and the expiratory reserve volume decrease, resulting in an obligate reduction in functional residual capacity. During pregnancy, the vital ability remains the same. Because of the reduction in residual volume, total lung capacity is only slightly reduced. The reduction in residual volume has a minor impact on total lung capacity. The tidal volume is raised, resulting in an increase in minute volume [4]. Early in pregnancy, both renal plasma flow and glomerular filtration rate rise. The increase in glomerular filtration rate reaches 50%, lowering serum creatinine to 0.8 mg/dL, the upper limit of average. Only a few changes in the gastrointestinal tract during pregnancy are essential in terms of critical care. The time it takes for the stomach to clear and the chance of aspiration that comes with general anaesthesia are both increased during labour. Placental development may cause a significant increase in alkaline phosphatase, but this does not mean hepatic obstruction. Gallbladder stasis can lead to increased stone formation.

The liver is the primary source of net endogenous glucose development while not pregnant. Fasting glucose levels in pregnant women decline as the pregnancy progresses [5]. GDM is characterised as the presence of glucose concentrations in pregnant women that are at the upper end of the population range for glucose and are first observed during pregnancy [6]. Insulin sensitivity decreases overall during pregnancy. Maternal insulin sensitivity, characterised as a decrease in the glucose infusion rate during the euglycemic hyperinsulinemic clamp to maintain 90 mg/dL, decreases in lean women during early pregnancy [7]. Since lean women are more likely to begin their pregnancies with greater insulin sensitivity than obese women, the increases in insulin concentration are more pronounced in lean women [8]. During pregnancy, healthy pregnant women's adipose tissue stores increase significantly. The mother and foetus can easily obtain calories from the subcutaneous stores, particularly during late pregnancy and lactation. Increases in visceral fat can be linked to decreased insulin sensitivity during late pregnancy [9].

In their research, Das and Sarka found that pregnant women faced a variety of difficulties when seeking health information, including inadequate hospital treatment, long wait times, anxiety and shame about discussing pregnancy with a physician, and a lack of time [10]. There are many discomforts that occur during pregnancy. Morning sickness, headache and backache, bladder and bowel changes, changes in hair and skin colour, indigestion and heartburn, leg cramps and swelling, vaginal thrush and discharge are the few common complications facing during pregnancy. As a result, the aim of this study was to describe the difficulties in obtaining health information and the measures to overcome the discomfort during pregnancy.

2. Materials and methods

Research articles for this review were searched by using the keywords "pregnancy", health issues", "measures to overcome", "challenges". The following were used as exclusion criteria: 1) the subject was unrelated to the study's goal; 2) there was no abstract available; 3) The research was limited to a single medical issue involving pregnancy in older women. 4) The report dealt with postpartum and maternity issues; and 5) the full research paper was not easily accessible. We looked for original research papers that were written in English and reported on studies that were performed using qualitative or quantitative methods. The current research did not include any other review papers. There were studies that looked at the health problems that women face during pregnancy were included in this review article.

3. Dental problems

According to previous literature, pregnant women's dental health care demands differ dramatically from those of the general population. The most frequent oral health concerns during pregnancy include periodontal disease, Xerostomia, halitosis, and tooth movement. During pregnancy, the hormonal balance of pregnant women alters. Because the placenta produces increased levels of oestrogen and progesterone during pregnancy, several tissues endure modifications. Increased sensitivity to irritations arises in the gingiva during this time [11]. Low vitamin C levels are thought to be another cause of this condition. When compared to mothers with healthy periodontium, mothers with attachment loss have an increased risk of giving birth to babies with low birth weight [12]. Tooth decay is more common among pregnant women for a variety of reasons, including increased acidity in the mouth, sweet food demands, and a lack of attention to oral health. Vomiting can have a severe impact on oral hygiene and induce degradation of the mother enamel layer [13]. Due to the effect of pregnancy hormones, pregnant women bleed more easily and may postpone brushing their teeth and it leads to an increase in bacterial plaque [14]. Due to diminished flow of saliva, caries are more likely to develop at this time. Pregnancy oral tumour is indistinguishable from pyogenic granuloma and occurs in up to 5% of pregnancies. Increased progesterone, in combination with local irritants and microorganisms, causes this vascular lesion [15]. With a prevalence of 60 to 75 percent, gingivitis is the most frequent dental illness among pregnant women. A severe aggravation of preexisting gingivitis occurs in around half of all pregnant women [16]. Researchers discovered very few oral bacteria in the amniotic fluid and placenta of women who had preterm labour with periodontitis in one investigation [17]. PGE2 production reduces placental blood flow, resulting in placental necrosis and intrauterine growth restriction [18]. Salivary oestrogen levels are greater in women who are expecting preterm babies than in women who are expecting full-term babies. Salivary oestrogen promotes oral mucosa proliferation and desquamation, as well as a rise in subgingival crevicular fluid levels. Desquamating cells offer a favourable environment for bacterial growth by supplying nutrients, hence preventing infection [19].

3.1 Management

Oral acid exposure is reduced through dietary and lifestyle changes, as well as the use of antiemetics, antacids, or both. Acid can be neutralised by rinsing the mouth with a teaspoon of baking soda in a cup of water after vomiting [20]. To lessen the risk of enamel damage, pregnant women should be encouraged to avoid brushing their teeth shortly after vomiting and to brush with a toothbrush with soft bristles when they do. Fluoride mouthwash can protect teeth that have been eroded or are sensitive. Proper dental hygiene can help women with previous periodontal disease lower the risk of recurrence or worsening disease during pregnancy. Education, clear communication, and the creation of continuing collaborative relationships can help physicians and dentists solve this dilemma. Physicians and dental colleagues can communicate information about the safety of dental treatment during pregnancy [21]. There is a link between plaque accumulation and caries prevalence during pregnancy and preventive maintenance methods. Mouthwashes or warm salty water should be gargled. Gums are relaxed and gum sensitivity is reduced by drinking warm salty water [22]. During this time, women can maintain their oral health by taking the required precautions, preventing potentially irreversible tooth disorders.

4. Hypertension

The mother's cardiovascular physiology adapts significantly as a result of the hormonal changes that occur during pregnancy [23]. Oestrogen, progesterone, and relaxin levels rise early in the first trimester, resulting in systemic vasodilation [24]. The RAAS is activated to promote salt and water retention, resulting in an increase in plasma volume. When this is paired with an increase in ventricular wall mass, it results in greater stroke volume. During pregnancy, the combination of increased stroke volume and tachycardia causes an increase in cardiac output, which compensates for the decrease in vascular resistance in order to keep blood pressure high enough for mother and placental perfusion [25]. The increased volume load in the heart causes left ventricular hypertrophy, which is proportional to the increased cardiac labour necessary to accomplish the increased cardiac output [26]. Some changes in the systemic hemodynamics of pregnant women who are predisposed to hypertension may occur before the condition manifests itself clinically. A systolic blood pressure of 160 mmHg or a diastolic blood pressure of 110 mmHg, or both, indicates severe preeclampsia in pregnancy. Eclampsia is a severe form of pregnancy-induced hypertension that affects one in every 1,600 pregnancies and appears at the end of the pregnancy [27]. When compared to singleton pregnancies, twin pregnancies had more than three times the risk of developing hypertension during pregnancy [28]. Preeclamptic patients have lower renin levels than non-pregnant women, although they are still significantly higher than non-pregnant women. Because most preeclamptic individuals have a somewhat reduced plasma volume, maintaining relatively high levels of these hormones may be necessary [29].

Preeclampsia is the pathophysiology of de novo hypertension and proteinuria in pregnancy. The delivery of the placenta frequently triggers the remission of preeclampsia's acute clinical symptoms, implying that the placenta plays a key role in the disease's pathophysiology. The placenta undergoes substantial blood supply throughout normal pregnancy to allow circulation between the foetus and the mother [30]. The pathogenesis of preeclampsia has long been focused on altered uteroplacental blood flow. Relaxin is a hormone secreted more during pregnancy which acts as vasodilation. According to Jeyabalan et al., low first trimester relaxin concentrations were linked to an increased risk of preeclampsia [31].

4.1 Management

For non-severe hypertension in pregnancy, oral labetalol is a first-line treatment [32]. Other beta-blockers, such as oxprenolol, are less thoroughly studied than labetalol, and it is used as a first-line treatment for non-severe hypertension in pregnancy [33]. In contrast, when oxprenolol was compared to methyldopa, the results and safety were found to be equal [34]. When mothers are exposed to calcium channel blockers during the first trimester, there is low teratogenicity [35]. Elsewhere in pregnancy, ACE inhibitors are still the first-line treatment for hypertension [36]. For non-severe hypertension, thiazide diuretics are considered second-line therapy.

5. Gestational diabetes (GDM)

The prevalence of gestational diabetes mellitus (GDM) is rising in lockstep with the rise in overweight and obesity among women of childbearing age. GDM-affected pregnancies increase the risk of caesarean and surgical vaginal delivery, macrosomia, neonatal hypoglycemia, and hyperbilirubinemia for both mother and child [37]. The onset of GDM is linked to a number of risk factors. Obesity, advanced maternal age, a significant family history of diabetes and belonging to an ethnic group are with a high prevalence of T2DM, polycystic ovarian syndrome, and chronic glucosuria. Because GDM usually starts in the late second trimester, when development is complete, congenital abnormalities do not occur at a higher rate in people with gestational diabetes. Because of the physiological, endocrine, and metabolic changes that occur throughout pregnancy in order to meet the fetus's constant nutritional and oxygen needs, a diabetogenic condition comparable to type 2 diabetes (T2D) develops, increasing insulin resistance, lowering insulin sensitivity, and thus increasing the demand for insulin [38]. As a result of the increased placental glucose transport, maternal hyperglycemia causes foetal hyperinsulinemia. Foetal macrosomia is caused by a high insulin level in the foetus, which accelerates growth [39]. Although glucose metabolism changes during pregnancy, tolerance occurs and there is no effect on the mother or the foetus when insulin production rises. There is a higher risk of foetal when there is an inappropriate response. When the output of the pancreatic b-cells does not match the insulin requirement of the tissues as a result of alterations in insulin resistance, abnormal glucose tolerance ensues [40]. Early in pregnancy, fasting blood glucose levels drop, and this trend continues throughout the pregnancy. Insulin sensitivity decreases as pregnancy progresses, reaching pre-gravid levels about 34–36 weeks of pregnancy [40, 41]. Increases in hepatic glucose production during pregnancy show that the insulin action deficiency also affects the liver. Placental loss of anti-insulin hormones such as human placental lactogen, cortisol, oestrogen, and progesterone causes insulin resistance after mid-pregnancy. Low FBS, a low kidney glucose threshold, and enhanced insulin production are all effects of these hormones [42]. Maternal tissues become increasingly insulin resistant during pregnancy. This is thought to be produced in part by placental hormones and in part by unknown obesity and pregnancy-related variables. The main locations for glucose disposal throughout the body are skeletal muscle and adipose tissue. Insulin-mediated whole-body glucose elimination declines by 50% during pregnancy, and the woman must raise her insulin output by 200–250 percent to maintain a euglycemic condition [43]. Even while most women revert to a euglycaemic state immediately after delivery, women who have had GDM have a significantly higher chance of developing T2DM [44]. The biochemical relationship between GDM and T2DM is still unknown. Insulin resistance and/or aberrant insulin production define both illnesses [45]. Multiple potential protein indicators for later GDM have been discovered through proteomic screening in early pregnancy, including a cluster linked with insulin production, binding, resistance, and signalling [46]. An oral glucose tolerance test (OGTT) is usually used to identify GDM during 24–28 weeks of pregnancy. Because most of the physiologic insulin resistance of pregnancy will be firmly established, this timeframe has traditionally been favoured for routine GDM diagnosis. Another important difference in GDM testing techniques around the world is the ongoing debate over whether testing should be universal (for all pregnant women) or targeted solely for women with risk factors linked to a higher probability of a positive result.

5.1 Management

Preventive interventions are needed to avoid the undesired consequences of obesity and hyperglycemia during pregnancy, given the global rise in obesity and the resulting increase in GDM [38, 47]. In roughly 70 to 85 percent of women with diagnosed GDM, lifestyle changes are enough to meet glycemic objectives [48]. Dietary counselling, in combination with physical activity and blood glucose self-monitoring, is the major intervention indicated for GDM [49]. A lower-carbohydrate diet with more animal protein and fat enhanced the risk of type 2 diabetes. As a result, it's possible that the diet that's best for treating GDM in women is not the best long-term diet [50]. Other nutritional treatments, such as probiotics and vitamin supplements, have gained popularity, but there is not enough data to suggest their widespread usage [51]. Insulin therapy is the preferred treatment because it does not cross the placenta and is thus deemed safe for the foetus. Metformin therapy was deemed safe and effective, and the women preferred it for insulin treatment [52]. Another study states that Metformin and sulfonylurea have been increasingly and safely used in the treatment of GDM [53]. In diabetic pregnant women with vitamin D deficiency/insufficiency, vitamin D administration can lower the chance of developing GDM and/or improve glycemic control [54]. Vitamin D regulates intracellular calcium to promote insulin production and attenuates insulin resistance by acting directly on pancreatic beta cells via the development of vitamin D receptors and the enzyme 25(OH)D-1-alfa-hydroxylase [55]. Furthermore, recent evidence from a large prospective trial suggests that increased physical activity may help reduce the risk of T2DM progression [56]. Exercise activities did not have a significant influence on the overall incidence of GDM in obese or overweight pregnant women, but when the effect measure was taken into account, the incidence of GDM was 24 percent lower in that group [57]. The following five components of guideline content were examined: GDM diagnosis, prenatal care, intrapartum care, neonatal care, and postpartum care. The majority of the suggestions in the guidelines were on prenatal care, particularly all types of therapy that could lower the risk of bad pregnancy outcomes due to uncontrolled blood sugar prior to conception [58]. The usage of information technology and digital platforms by diabetic pregnant women is fast rising around the world [59]. Telemedicine has been linked to high patient satisfaction since it allows for quick management of care across distances with fewer face-to-face physician appointments [60]. As a result, the use of e-platforms in the management of gestational diabetes shows encouraging results in terms of patient satisfaction and has no negative impact on pregnancy outcomes. Adequately powered RCTs are needed to assess whether such healthcare technologies are cost-effective or can help enhance care in urban or distant settings [61].

6. Gestational thrombocytopenia and anaemia

During pregnancy, several biological markers, particularly haematological, are physiologically altered. Biologists and doctors who are aware of these changes in the maternal body can screen for potential abnormalities. The haematological parameters must adjust in several ways, including providing vitamins and minerals for foetal haematopoiesis (iron, vitamin B12, folic acid), which can increase maternal anaemia, and preparing for birth bleeding, which is necessary to improve homeostasis [62]. The total blood volume increases by roughly 1.5 litres during pregnancy, primarily to meet the demands of the new vascular bed and to compensate for blood loss that occurs during birth [63]. At 6–12 weeks of pregnancy, the plasma volume expands by 10–15 percent. When maternal erythropoietin production rises, RBC mass rises as well, albeit at a slower rate than plasma volume, resulting in a drop in haemoglobin concentration. Dilutional anaemia is the result [64]. Haemodilution also contributes to a decrease in the rate of haematocrit (HCT) and haemoglobin (HGB), resulting in a false anaemia. Such a change is natural for pregnant women and demonstrates the adoption of a different threshold for the definition of pregnancy anaemia. The WHO defines anaemia in pregnancy as having a total circulating HGB concentration of less than 11 g/dl or an HCT of less than 33% at any point during the pregnancy. During pregnancy, RBC indices do not vary much. However, in an iron-replete woman, there is a slight rise in mean corpuscular volume (MCV) of around 4 fl, which peaks around 30–35 weeks gestation and does not indicate a vitamin B12 or folate shortage. The increased MCV can be explained by increased RBC production to fulfil the demands of pregnancy [65]. The haemoglobin concentration does not change until the 16th week of pregnancy, after which it falls steadily to the second trimester due to the expansion of plasma volume [66]. Haemodilution, or an increase in plasma volume greater than an increase in red cell mass, is the underlying cause of anaemia during pregnancy. This condition is also known as 'physiological anaemia of pregnancy' [67]. Because length is more stable than weight, haemoglobin demonstrated a positive connection with infant length but not with weight [68]. Haemoglobin and haematocrit increased on the first day after birth, decreased on the third and fifth days, and then began to rise again by day 42, achieving normal haemoglobin in non-pregnant women [69]. Because of the greater metabolic oxygen requirement, erythropoietin levels are 50 percent greater, which explains the mild bone marrow erythroid hyperplasia and enhanced reticulocyte count. A combination of a lowered maternal RBCs oxygen affinity from an enhanced 2,3 Diphosphoglycerate and a low maternal pCO2 results in enhanced oxygen transfer throughout the placenta [70].

Pregnancy causes an increase in white blood cell count, with the lowest limit of the reference range typically being 6,000/cumm. Leucocytosis occurs during pregnancy as a result of the physiologic stress that comes with being pregnant [71]. Throughout the first and second trimesters of pregnancy, lymphocyte count drops, then rises during the third trimester. Total leukocyte count levels rise significantly in the II and III trimesters, but there is no difference between pregnant and non-pregnant women in the I trimester. In the first trimester of pregnancy, non-anaemic women have a higher TLC count than anaemic women, but in the second and third trimesters, anaemic women have a higher TLC count than non-anaemic women [62]. During normal pregnancy, leukocytosis is caused by an enhanced inflammatory response, which can be caused by selective immunological tolerance, immunosuppression, and immunomodulation of the foetus [72]. During pregnancy, the ratio of monocytes to lymphocytes rises dramatically. During pregnancy, however, eosinophil and basophil numbers do not alter appreciably [73]. The neutrophil count starts to rise in the second month of pregnancy and reaches a plateau in the second or third trimester, when total white blood cell counts range from 9,000 to 15,000 cells per microliter.

In 7–8 percent of all pregnancies, gestational thrombocytopenia occurs. Due to rapid degradation, platelet counts are slightly lower which results in younger, bigger platelets present in pregnancy. The majority of thrombocytopenia in pregnancy is caused by increased blood loss [74]. Although the average platelet count falls monotonically during pregnancy, platelet aggregation increases, notably during the last 8 weeks of pregnancy [75]. The decline in the quantity of circulating platelets during pregnancy has been attributed to increased platelet consumption as well as a shorter life span in the uteroplacental circulation [76]. As the pregnancy progresses, the platelet volume distribution width widens dramatically and continually. As a result, as pregnancy progresses, the mean platelet volume becomes an insensitive indicator of platelet size.

Primary immune thrombocytopenia (ITP) affects about 3% of women who are thrombocytopenic at delivery. It occurs in 1/1000–1/10 000 pregnancies [77]. Two-thirds of women with ITP have pre-existing disease, according to most studies, and one-third are diagnosed for the first time during pregnancy [78]. The pathophysiological mechanism of thrombotic thrombocytopenic purpura (TTP) is thrombotic microangiopathy. Microangiopathic hemolytic anaemia, thrombocytopenia, fever, neurological signs, and renal impairment are all symptoms of TTP. Pregnancy is thought to be the trigger event in between 5 to 25% of TTP cases [79]. TTP occurs in the second trimester of pregnancy and occasionally in the postpartum period, although it is uncommon in the first trimester [80]. If TTP appears during the first trimester, regular plasma exchange may be able to maintain pregnancy.

6.1 Management

Preventing anaemia in pregnancy requires effective communication about diet and nutrition to all pregnant women. Most experts recommend regular iron supplementation during pregnancy since the extra demand for iron is typically unmet by a typical diet. Although iron supplementation recommendations vary by location, the CDC recommends that all pregnant women begin a 30 mg/day iron supplementation [81]. he average iron density in a typical Indian diet is 8.5 mg/1000 Kcal, with 13.3 and 5.3 percent iron absorption in pregnancy from a rice-based and wheat-based Indian diet, respectively [82]. Women can use smartphone applications to learn about their daily iron needs, the iron content of various foods, and how to track their dietary iron intake. We support the creation and use of such applications. For improved absorption, all pregnant women should be told to take oral iron on an empty stomach or 1 hour after meals, preferably with a vitamin C-rich product like orange juice or guava. Supplement 2 outlines the oral iron treatments that can be used during pregnancy [82, 83].

The choice of therapy is based on the urgency of the platelet increase, the duration of the increase, and any potential side effects, and should be determined on an individual basis for each patient. Platelets should be available on standby if the mother's platelet count remains low (50 109/l) around the time of delivery, but they are likely to be destroyed rapidly after infusion if due to an immune reaction, so they should be given in well-established rather than early labour if there are increased bleeding complications [84]. Given that there is no evidence that Caesarean delivery is safer for the foetus with thrombocytopenia than a simple vaginal delivery, which is usually safer than caesarean for the mother, the mode of delivery should be decided on obstetric concerns. Treatment may be required just during the later part of the third trimester to boost the platelet level before epidural anaesthesia or C section section if the individual is asymptomatic and the platelet count is more than $20*10^9/L$ [85]. Depending on the platelet level and stability, general measures such as avoiding aspirin, nonsteroidal anti-inflammatory medications, and intramuscular injections might be explored. Because low-dose aspirin is now commonly administered in pregnancy for a variety of reasons, it should not be avoided unless the risk of bleeding is significant. Prednisone at a low dose or intravenous immunoglobulin, or both, are viable alternatives in these circumstances. In symptomatic pregnant ITP patients or if the platelet count is less than standard level, other therapeutic options are available. When combined with intravenous immunoglobulin, a large dose of steroids can be employed [86]. Corticosteroids and intravenous IVIG are the most common treatments for maternal ITP [87].

7. Conclusion

When it came to getting health information, pregnant women faced personal, societal, and structural challenges. As a result, legislators and health planners should remove barriers, promote self-care, and improve the quality of life for pregnant women, ultimately improving their health. Pregnancy issues such as gestational diabetes mellitus, hypertension, preeclampsia, caesarean birth, and postpartum weight retention are all more likely in overweight and obese women. More research into the link between nutritional advancements and the rising prevalence of GDM in the developing world is needed. Iron supplementation has been linked to glucose dysregulation and hypertension in mid-pregnancy; its effectiveness and potential risks should be carefully considered.

Acknowledgements

I would like to thank Saveetha Institute of Medical and Technical Sciences for giving me this opportunity to carry out the research work.

Funding Support

This study received no specific support from public, private, or non-profit funding bodies.

Conflict of interest

No potential conflict of interest relevant to this article was reported.

Author details

Gayatri Devi Ramalingam[1*], Saravana Kumar Sampath[2] and Jothi Priya Amirtham[1]

1 Department of Physiology, Saveetha Dental College, SIMATS, Chennai, Tamil Nadu, India

2 Department of Anatomy, SEGI University, Malaysia

*Address all correspondence to: gayatri.physio88@gmail.com; dr.sharan_anatomist@yahoo.com

References

[1] Jung J, Horta H, Yonezawa A. Researching Higher Education in Asia: History, Development and Future. Springer; 2017. 366 p.

[2] Pritchard JA. Changes in the Blood Volume During Pregnancy and Delivery [Internet]. Vol. 26, Anesthesiology. 1965. p. 393-9. Available from: http://dx.doi.org/10.1097/00000542-196507000-00004

[3] Toglia MR, Weg JG. Venous Thromboembolism during Pregnancy [Internet]. Vol. 335, New England Journal of Medicine. 1996. p. 108-14. Available from: http://dx.doi.org/10.1056/nejm199607113350207

[4] Website.

[5] Website.

[6] Catalano PM, Huston L, Amini SB, Kalhan SC. Longitudinal changes in glucose metabolism during pregnancy in obese women with normal glucose tolerance and gestational diabetes mellitus [Internet]. Vol. 180, American Journal of Obstetrics and Gynecology. 1999. p. 903-16. Available from: http://dx.doi.org/10.1016/s0002-9378(99)70662-9

[7] Catalano PM, Tyzbir ED, Wolfe RR, Calles J, Roman NM, Amini SB, et al. Carbohydrate metabolism during pregnancy in control subjects and women with gestational diabetes [Internet]. Vol. 264, American Journal of Physiology-Endocrinology and Metabolism. 1993. p. E60-7. Available from: http://dx.doi.org/10.1152/ajpendo.1993.264.1.e60

[8] Lain KY, Catalano PM. Metabolic changes in pregnancy. Clin Obstet Gynecol. 2007 Dec;50(4):938-948.

[9] Kitzmiller J, Jovanovic L, Brown F, Coustan D. Managing Preexisting Diabetes and Pregnancy: Technical Reviews and Consensus Recommendations for Care. American Diabetes Association; 2008. 852 p.

[10] Das A, Sarkar M. Pregnancy-related health information-seeking behaviors among rural pregnant women in India: validating the Wilson model in the Indian context. Yale J Biol Med. 2014 Sep;87(3):251-262.

[11] Dörtbudak O, Eberhardt R, Ulm M, Persson GR. Periodontitis, a marker of risk in pregnancy for preterm birth. J Clin Periodontol. 2005 Jan;32(1):45-52.

[12] Offenbacher S. Maternal Periodontal Infections, Prematurity, and Growth Restriction [Internet]. Vol. 47, Clinical Obstetrics and Gynecology. 2004. p. 808-21. Available from: http://dx.doi.org/10.1097/01.grf.0000141894.85221.f7

[13] Silk H, Douglass AB, Maier R, Clark M, Deutchman M, Douglass J, et al. Smiles for Life National Oral Health Curriculum: Module 5. Oral Health in Pregnancy [Internet]. Vol. 8, MedEdPORTAL. 2012. Available from: http://dx.doi.org/10.15766/mep_2374-8265.9259

[14] Website [Internet]. [cited 2021 May 26]. Available from: https://doi.org/10.4103/0976-9668.166124

[15] Sills ES, Zegarelli DJ, Hoschander MM, Strider WE. Clinical diagnosis and management of hormonally responsive oral pregnancy tumor (pyogenic granuloma). J Reprod Med. 1996 Jul;41(7):467-470.

[16] Website [Internet]. [cited 2021 May 26]. Available from: American Dental Association Council on Access, Prevention and Interprofessional Relations. Women's oral health issues. American Dental Association, 2006. http://www.ada.org/prof/resources/

topics/healthcare_womens.pdf. Accessed August 1, 2007.

[17] Goepfert AR, Jeffcoat MK, Andrews WW, Faye-Petersen O, Cliver SP, Goldenberg RL, et al. Periodontal Disease and Upper Genital Tract Inflammation in Early Spontaneous Preterm Birth [Internet]. Vol. 104, Obstetrics & Gynecology. 2004. p. 777-83. Available from: http://dx.doi.org/10.1097/01.aog.0000139836.47777.6d

[18] Offenbacher S, Lieff S, Boggess KA, Murtha AP, Madianos PN, Champagne CME, et al. Maternal Periodontitis and Prematurity. Part I: Obstetric Outcome of Prematurity and Growth Restriction [Internet]. Vol. 6, Annals of Periodontology. 2001. p. 164-74. Available from: http://dx.doi.org/10.1902/annals.2001.6.1.164

[19] Lopez BC, Chaveli Lopez B, Perez MGS, Jimenez Soriano Y. Dental considerations in pregnancy and menopause [Internet]. Journal of Clinical and Experimental Dentistry. 2011. p. e135-44. Available from: http://dx.doi.org/10.4317/jced.3.e135

[20] Wright GZ, Kupietzky A. Behavior Management in Dentistry for Children. John Wiley & Sons; 2014. 264 p.

[21] Livingston HM, Mark Livingston H, Dellinger TM, Holder R. Considerations in the management of the pregnant patient [Internet]. Vol. 18, Special Care in Dentistry. 1998. p. 183-8. Available from: http://dx.doi.org/10.1111/j.1754-4505.1998.tb01737.x

[22] Zanata RL, Navarro MF de L, Pereira JC, Franco EB, Lauris JRP, Barbosa SH. Effect of caries preventive measures directed to expectant mothers on caries experience in their children. Braz Dent J. 2003 Oct 3;14(2):75-81.

[23] Sanghavi M, Rutherford JD. Cardiovascular Physiology of Pregnancy [Internet]. Vol. 130, Circulation. 2014. p. 1003-8. Available from: http://dx.doi.org/10.1161/circulationaha.114.009029

[24] Kodogo V, Azibani F, Sliwa K. Role of pregnancy hormones and hormonal interaction on the maternal cardiovascular system: a literature review. Clin Res Cardiol. 2019 Aug;108(8):831-846.

[25] Ngene NC, Moodley J. Physiology of blood pressure relevant to managing hypertension in pregnancy. J Matern Fetal Neonatal Med. 2019 Apr;32(8):1368-1377.

[26] Simmons LA, Gillin AG, Jeremy RW. Structural and functional changes in left ventricle during normotensive and preeclamptic pregnancy [Internet]. Vol. 283, American Journal of Physiology-Heart and Circulatory Physiology. 2002. p. H1627-33. Available from: http://dx.doi.org/10.1152/ajpheart.00966.2001

[27] L. PK, Professor A, Permi HS, V. MS, Guruprasad Y, Professor A, et al. Study of Biochemical Parameters in Pregnancy Induced Hypertension (PIH) [Internet]. Vol. 5, Indian Journal of Pathology: Research and Practice. 2016. p. 191-4. Available from: http://dx.doi.org/10.21088/ijprp.2278.148x.5216.21

[28] Tessema GA, Tekeste A, Ayele TA. Preeclampsia and associated factors among pregnant women attending antenatal care in Dessie referral hospital, Northeast Ethiopia: a hospital-based study [Internet]. Vol. 15, BMC Pregnancy and Childbirth. 2015. Available from: http://dx.doi.org/10.1186/s12884-015-0502-7

[29] Luft FC, Eileen D. M. Gallery, Lindheimer MD. Normal and Abnormal Volume Homeostasis [Internet]. Chesley's Hypertensive Disorders in Pregnancy. 2009. p. 269-85. Available from: http://dx.doi.org/10.1016/b978-0-12-374213-1.00015-x

[30] Agarwal I, Ananth Karumanchi S. Preeclampsia and the anti-angiogenic state [Internet]. Vol. 1, Pregnancy Hypertension: An International Journal of Women's Cardiovascular Health. 2011. p. 17-21. Available from: http://dx.doi.org/10.1016/j.preghy.2010.10.007

[31] Tregear GW, Ivell R, Bathgate RA, Wade JD. Relaxin 2000. Springer Science & Business Media; 2001. 460 p.

[32] Tranquilli AL, Dekker G, Magee L, Roberts J, Sibai BM, Steyn W, et al. The classification, diagnosis and management of the hypertensive disorders of pregnancy: A revised statement from the ISSHP [Internet]. Vol. 4, Pregnancy Hypertension: An International Journal of Women's Cardiovascular Health. 2014. p. 97-104. Available from: http://dx.doi.org/10.1016/j.preghy.2014.02.001

[33] Redman CWG. Hypertension in pregnancy: the NICE guidelines [Internet]. Vol. 97, Heart. 2011. p. 1967-9. Available from: http://dx.doi.org/10.1136/heartjnl-2011-300949

[34] Fidler J, Smith V, Fayers P, De Swiet M. Randomised controlled comparative study of methyldopa and oxprenolol in treatment of hypertension in pregnancy [Internet]. Vol. 286, BMJ. 1983. p. 1927-30. Available from: http://dx.doi.org/10.1136/bmj.286.6382.1927

[35] Magee LA, Schick B, Donnenfeld AE, Sage SR, Conover B, Cook L, et al. The safety of calcium channel blockers in human pregnancy: a prospective, multicenter cohort study. Am J Obstet Gynecol. 1996 Mar;174(3):823-828.

[36] Guideline for the Diagnosis and Management of Hypertension in Adults. 2016. 74 p.

[37] Catalano PM, Ehrenberg HM. Review article: The short- and long-term implications of maternal obesity on the mother and her offspring [Internet]. Vol. 113, BJOG: An International Journal of Obstetrics & Gynaecology. 2006. p. 1126-33. Available from: http://dx.doi.org/10.1111/j.1471-0528.2006.00989.x

[38] Mottola MF, Artal R. Role of Exercise in Reducing Gestational Diabetes Mellitus [Internet]. Vol. 59, Clinical Obstetrics & Gynecology. 2016. p. 620-8. Available from: http://dx.doi.org/10.1097/grf.0000000000000211

[39] The Pregnant Diabetic and Her Newborn. Problems and Management [Internet]. Vol. 43, Archives of Disease in Childhood. 1968. p. 391-391. Available from: http://dx.doi.org/10.1136/adc.43.229.391-a

[40] Kim C, Ferrara A. Gestational Diabetes During and After Pregnancy. Springer Science & Business Media; 2010. 394 p.

[41] Catalano PM, Tyzbir ED, Roman NM, Amini SB, Sims EAH. Longitudinal changes in insulin release and insulin resistance in nonobese pregnant women [Internet]. Vol. 165, American Journal of Obstetrics and Gynecology. 1991. p. 1667-72. Available from: http://dx.doi.org/10.1016/0002-9378(91)90012-g

[42] A review article- gestational diabetes mellitus. Int J Endocrinol Metab. 2019 Feb 7;7(1):62-5.

[43] Barbour LA, McCurdy CE, Hernandez TL, Kirwan JP, Catalano PM, Friedman JE. Cellular Mechanisms for Insulin Resistance in Normal Pregnancy and Gestational Diabetes [Internet]. Vol. 30, Diabetes Care. 2007. p. S112-9. Available from: http://dx.doi.org/10.2337/dc07-s202

[44] Bellamy L, Casas J-P, Hingorani AD, Williams D. Type 2 diabetes mellitus after gestational diabetes: a systematic review and meta-analysis [Internet].

Vol. 373, The Lancet. 2009. p. 1773-9. Available from: http://dx.doi.org/10.1016/s0140-6736(09)60731-5

[45] Lauenborg J, Grarup N, Damm P, Borch-Johnsen K, Jørgensen T, Pedersen O, et al. Common type 2 diabetes risk gene variants associate with gestational diabetes. J Clin Endocrinol Metab. 2009 Jan;94(1):145-150.

[46] Zhou T, Huang L, Wang M, Chen D, Chen Z, Jiang S-W. A Critical Review of Proteomic Studies in Gestational Diabetes Mellitus. J Diabetes Res. 2020 Jul 14;2020:6450352.

[47] Bain E, Crane M, Tieu J, Han S, Crowther CA, Middleton P. Diet and exercise interventions for preventing gestational diabetes mellitus [Internet]. Cochrane Database of Systematic Reviews. 2015. Available from: http://dx.doi.org/10.1002/14651858.cd010443.pub2

[48] Association AD, American Diabetes Association. 13. Management of Diabetes in Pregnancy:Standards of Medical Care in Diabetes—2018 [Internet]. Vol. 41, Diabetes Care. 2018. p. S137-43. Available from: http://dx.doi.org/10.2337/dc18-s013

[49] Lapolla A, Fedele D, Dalfra. Management of gestational diabetes mellitus [Internet]. Vol. 2, Diabetes, Metabolic Syndrome and Obesity: Targets and Therapy. 2009. p. 73-82. Available from: http://dx.doi.org/10.2147/dmso.s3407

[50] Bao W, Li S, Chavarro JE, Tobias DK, Zhu Y, Hu FB, et al. Low Carbohydrate–Diet Scores and Long-term Risk of Type 2 Diabetes Among Women With a History of Gestational Diabetes Mellitus: A Prospective Cohort Study [Internet]. Vol. 39, Diabetes Care. 2016. p. 43-9. Available from: http://dx.doi.org/10.2337/dc15-1642

[51] Dolatkhah N, Hajifaraji M, Abbasalizadeh F, Aghamohammadzadeh N, Mehrabi Y, Abbasi MM. Is there a value for probiotic supplements in gestational diabetes mellitus? A randomized clinical trial [Internet]. Vol. 33, Journal of Health, Population and Nutrition. 2015. Available from: http://dx.doi.org/10.1186/s41043-015-0034-9

[52] Rowan JA, Hague WM, Gao W, Battin MR, Peter Moore M. Metformin versus Insulin for the Treatment of Gestational Diabetes [Internet]. Vol. 358, New England Journal of Medicine. 2008. p. 2003-15. Available from: http://dx.doi.org/10.1056/nejmoa0707193

[53] Dhulkotia JS, Ola B, Fraser R, Farrell T. Oral hypoglycemic agents vs insulin in management of gestational diabetes: a systematic review and metaanalysis. Am J Obstet Gynecol. 2010 Nov;203(5):457.e1-9.

[54] Poel YHM, Hummel P, Lips P, Stam F, van der Ploeg T, Simsek S. Vitamin D and gestational diabetes: a systematic review and meta-analysis. Eur J Intern Med. 2012 Jul;23(5):465-469.

[55] Alvarez JA, Ashraf A. Role of vitamin d in insulin secretion and insulin sensitivity for glucose homeostasis. Int J Endocrinol. 2010;2010:351385.

[56] Bao W, Tobias DK, Bowers K, Chavarro J, Vaag A, Grunnet LG, et al. Physical activity and sedentary behaviors associated with risk of progression from gestational diabetes mellitus to type 2 diabetes mellitus: a prospective cohort study. JAMA Intern Med. 2014 Jul;174(7):1047-1055.

[57] Nasiri-Amiri F, Sepidarkish M, Shirvani MA, Habibipour P, Tabari NSM. The effect of exercise on the prevention of gestational diabetes in obese and overweight pregnant women:

a systematic review and meta-analysis. Diabetol Metab Syndr. 2019 Aug 27;11:72.

[58] Mahmud M, Mazza D. Preconception care of women with diabetes: a review of current guideline recommendations. BMC Womens Health. 2010 Jan 31;10:5.

[59] Diabetes Canada Clinical Practice Guidelines Expert Committee, Feig DS, Berger H, Donovan L, Godbout A, Kader T, et al. Diabetes and Pregnancy. Can J Diabetes. 2018 Apr;42 Suppl 1:S255-82.

[60] Ivey TL, Hughes D, Dajani NK, Magann EF. Antenatal management of at-risk pregnancies from a distance. Aust N Z J Obstet Gynaecol. 2015 Feb;55(1):87-89.

[61] Mitric C, Desilets J, Brown RN. Recent advances in the antepartum management of diabetes. F1000Res. 2019 May 8;8(622):622.

[62] Mohamed A, Hamza K, Babker A. Physiological changes in some hematological and coagulation profile among Sudanese healthy pregnant women [Internet]. Vol. 5, International Journal of Medical Science and Public Health. 2016. p. 525. Available from: http://dx.doi.org/10.5455/ijmsph.2016.30092015149

[63] Ramsay M. Normal hematological changes during pregnancy and the puerperium [Internet]. The Obstetric Hematology Manual. p. 3-12. Available from: http://dx.doi.org/10.1017/cbo9780511676451.002

[64] Bernstein IM, Ziegler W, Badger GJ. Plasma Volume Expansion in Early Pregnancy [Internet]. Vol. 97, Obstetrics & Gynecology. 2001. p. 669-72. Available from: http://dx.doi.org/10.1097/00006250-200105000-00005

[65] Taylor DJ, Lind T. Red cell mass during and after normal pregnancy. Br J Obstet Gynaecol. 1979 May;86(5):364-370.

[66] Micronutrient Initiative, Gallego EB, International Development Research Centre (Canada). Severe Anemia in Pregnancy: Report of a Workshop Held at the Institute of Child and Mother Health in Dhaka, Bangladesh. L'Initiative micronutriments = Micronutrient Initiative; 2000. 31 p.

[67] P S, Sharma P, Research Scholar, Department of Home Science, University of Rajasthan, Jaipur. Hematological profile of anemic pregnant women attending antenatal hospital [Internet]. Vol. 1, IOSR Journal of Nursing and Health Science. 2013. p. 11-5. Available from: http://dx.doi.org/10.9790/1959-0141115

[68] Weerd S de, de Weerd S, Steegers-Theunissen RPM, de Boo TM, Thomas CMG, Steegers EAP. Maternal periconceptional biochemical and hematological parameters, vitamin profiles and pregnancy outcome [Internet]. Vol. 57, European Journal of Clinical Nutrition. 2003. p. 1128-34. Available from: http://dx.doi.org/10.1038/sj.ejcn.1601654

[69] Ramakers C, Van Der WOUDE DAA, Verzijl JM, Pijnenborg JMA, Van WIJK EM. An added value for the hemoglobin content in reticulocytes (CHr) and the mean corpuscular volume (MCV) in the diagnosis of iron deficiency in postpartum anemic women [Internet]. Vol. 34, International Journal of Laboratory Hematology. 2012. p. 510-6. Available from: http://dx.doi.org/10.1111/j.1751-553x.2012.01423.x

[70] Madsen H, Ditzel J. Red cell 2,3-diphosphoglycerate and hemoglobin--oxygen affinity during

normal pregnancy. Acta Obstet Gynecol Scand. 1984;63(5):399-402.

[71] Akinlaja O. Hematological Changes in Pregnancy - The Preparation for Intrapartum Blood Loss [Internet]. Vol. 4, Obstetrics & Gynecology International Journal. 2016. Available from: http://dx.doi.org/10.15406/ogij.2016.04.00109

[72] Osonuga IO, Osonuga OA, Onadeko AA, Osonuga A, Osonuga AA. Hematological profile of pregnant women in southwest of Nigeria [Internet]. Vol. 1, Asian Pacific Journal of Tropical Disease. 2011. p. 232-4. Available from: http://dx.doi.org/10.1016/s2222-1808(11)60036-4

[73] Edelstam G, Löwbeer C, Kral G, Gustafsson SA, Venge P. New reference values for routine blood samples and human neutrophilic lipocalin during third-trimester pregnancy. Scand J Clin Lab Invest. 2001;61(8):583-592.

[74] Eledo BO. Evaluation of Some Haematological Parameters Among Post-menopausal Women in Bayelsa State, Nigeria: A Case Study of Patients Attending Federal Medical Centre, Yenagoa [Internet]. Vol. 2, American Journal of Laboratory Medicine. 2017. p. 132. Available from: http://dx.doi.org/10.11648/j.ajlm.20170206.14

[75] Fay RA, Hughes AO, Farron NT. Platelets in pregnancy: hyperdestruction in pregnancy. Obstet Gynecol. 1983 Feb;61(2):238-240.

[76] Ahmed Y, Van Iddekinge B, Paul C, Sullivan MHF, Elder MG. Retrospective analysis of platelet numbers and volumes in normal pregnancy and in pre-eclampsia [Internet]. Vol. 43, International Journal of Gynecology & Obstetrics. 1993. p. 230-230. Available from: http://dx.doi.org/10.1016/0020-7292(93)90342-t

[77] Gill KK, Kelton JG. Management of idiopathic thrombocytopenic purpura in pregnancy [Internet]. Vol. 37, Seminars in Hematology. 2000. p. 275-89. Available from: http://dx.doi.org/10.1053/shem.2000.8960

[78] Webert KE, Mittal R, Sigouin C, Heddle NM, Kelton JG. A retrospective 11-year analysis of obstetric patients with idiopathic thrombocytopenic purpura. Blood. 2003 Dec 15;102(13):4306-4311.

[79] Vesely SK, Li X, McMinn JR, Terrell DR, George JN. Pregnancy outcomes after recovery from thrombotic thrombocytopenic purpura-hemolytic uremic syndrome [Internet]. Vol. 44, Transfusion. 2004. p. 1149-58. Available from: http://dx.doi.org/10.1111/j.1537-2995.2004.03422.x

[80] Scully M, Hunt BJ, Benjamin S, Liesner R, Rose P, Peyvandi F, et al. Guidelines on the diagnosis and management of thrombotic thrombocytopenic purpura and other thrombotic microangiopathics [Internet]. Vol. 158, British Journal of Haematology. 2012. p. 323-35. Available from: http://dx.doi.org/10.1111/j.1365-2141.2012.09167.x

[81] Pavord S, Myers B, Robinson S, Allard S, Strong J, Oppenheimer C, et al. UK guidelines on the management of iron deficiency in pregnancy. Br J Haematol. 2012 Mar;156(5):588-600.

[82] Bothwell TH. Iron requirements in pregnancy and strategies to meet them [Internet]. Vol. 72, The American Journal of Clinical Nutrition. 2000. p. 257S – 264S. Available from: http://dx.doi.org/10.1093/ajcn/72.1.257s

[83] Jacob A. Medical Disorders Associated with Pregnancy [Internet]. A Comprehensive Textbook of Midwifery. 2008. p. 335-335. Available from: http://dx.doi.org/10.5005/jp/books/10008_29

[84] Myers B. Diagnosis and management of maternal thrombocytopenia in pregnancy [Internet]. Vol. 158, British Journal of Haematology. 2012. p. 3-15. Available from: http://dx.doi.org/10.1111/j.1365-2141.2012.09135.x

[85] Provan D, Stasi R, Newland AC, Blanchette VS, Bolton-Maggs P, Bussel JB, et al. International consensus report on the investigation and management of primary immune thrombocytopenia [Internet]. Vol. 115, Blood. 2010. p. 168-86. Available from: http://dx.doi.org/10.1182/blood-2009-06-225565

[86] Izak M, Bussel JB. Management of thrombocytopenia. F1000Prime Rep [Internet]. 2014 Jun 2 [cited 2021 May 28];6(45). Available from: https://facultyopinions.com/prime/reports/m/6/45/pdf

[87] Greaves M, Letsky EA. Guidelines on the investigation and management of thrombocytopenia in pregnancy and neonatal alloimmune thrombocytopenia [Internet]. Vol. 104, BJOG: An International Journal of Obstetrics and Gynaecology. 1997. p. 1108-1108. Available from: http://dx.doi.org/10.1111/j.1471-0528.1997.tb10931.x

Chapter 4

Premature Birth, Management, Complications

Panagiotis Tsikouras, Anastasia Bothou, Aggeliki Gerede, Ifigenia Apostolou, Fotini Gaitatzi, Dorelia Deuteraiou, Anna Chalkidou, Xanthoula Anthoulaki, Spyridon Michalopoulos, Georgios Dragoutsos, Ioannis Tsirkas, Irini Babageorgaka, Theopi Nalbanti, Natalia Sachnova, Alexios Alexiou, Constantinos Nikolettos, Apostolos Lazarou, Stefanos Zervoudis, Panagiotis Peitsidis and Nikolaos Nikolettos

Abstract

In recent years an increase in premature births (PB) rate has been noticed, as this pregnancy complication that still remain an important cause of perinatal morbidity and mortality, is multifactorial and prediction is not easy in many cases. There are many bibliographic data supporting the view that PB have also genetic predisposition. The trend of "recurrence" of PB in women as well as its increased frequency in ethnic groups suggests its association with genetic factors, either as such or as an interaction of genes and environment. Immunomodulatory molecules and receptors as well as polymorphisms of various genes and/or single nucleotides (single nucleotide polymorphisms, SNPs) now allow with advanced methods of Molecular Biology the identification of genes and proteins involved in the pathophysiology of PB. From the history of a pregnant woman, the main prognostic factor is a previous history of prematurity, while an ultrasound assessment of the cervix between 18 and 24 weeks is suggested, both in the developed and the developing world. According to the latest data, an effective method of successful prevention of premature birth has not been found. The main interventions suggested for the prevention of premature birth are the cervical cerclage, the use of cervical pessary, the use of progesterone orally, subcutaneously or transvaginally, and for treatment administration of tocolytic medication as an attempt to inhibit childbirth for at least 48 hours to make corticosteroids more effective. Despite the positive results in reducing mortality and morbidity of premature infants, the need for more research in the field of prevention, investigation of the genital code and the mechanism of initiation of preterm birth is important.

Keywords: preterm birth, predisponding factors, complications

1. Introduction

Premature birth defined as the onset of labor before the 37th week of pregnancy and is a clinical symptom that is accompanied by multiple pathogenetic causes. The etiology is multifactorial and complex. It is not a normal premature birth, but a distinct syndrome with specific characteristics [1–5]. Sometimes, the mother, the placenta and the fetus altogether are involved to a different degree. The exact mechanism is not known. Uterine cramps that cause premature birth are coordinated uterine contractions that cause progressive change (elimination and/or dilation) of the cervix before the 37th week of pregnancy. In contrast, premature contractions are rhythmic contractions of the uterus that do not cause a change in the cervix [1–5]. Specifically, in 1948, the World Health Organization (WHO) defined with the term "prematurity" the delivery of a newborn weighing <2500 g. The primary problem that arose was that it characterized a multitude of newborns with heterogeneous fetal development as premature. Therefore, in 1960 Battaglia and Lubchenco used measurements from a large population of newborns to establish the rules of fetal development.

Prematurity based on Birth Weight is divided into "low birth weight" infants <2500 g, "very low birth weight" infants <1500 g (approximately 1–1.5% of live births) and "extremely low birth weight" infants <1000 g (this category includes 0.7% of all live births).

Premature is the newborn that will be born at a gestational age less than the 37th week of pregnancy. Very premature is the newborn which will be born at a gestational age less than 32 weeks of gestation.

Premature birth is subdivided into automatic preterm birth as a consequence of premature contractions with an incidence of 35% of unknown etiology, a corresponding incidence of 25% resulting from premature rupture of membranes and in 25% of cases iatrogenic, as a consequence of medical or obstetric such as maternal hypertension, fetal development pathology and gestational bleeding, while in cases of multiple pregnancy the incidence rate is 15% [6–11].

2. Epidemiology

It contributes a large 75% to the formation of perinatal morbidity and mortality and it is estimated that about 50% of long-term neurological problems are related to prematurity. The incidence is between 10 and 12% over a period of about 15 years (1981–1996) and includes about 467,000 births in United States of America, compared to European developed countries in which the rates of prematurity are lower at 5–6%. Prematurity has gradually increased from 6–13% of all births and it is estimated that 13,000,000 premature babies are born per year worldwide [1–5].

The highest rate of 60% is observed in countries of South Asia and Central Africa while in African Americans it occurs with twice the frequency of 18% compared to Caucasians. It is generally and worldwide accepted that an embryo is viable for more than 20 weeks and in Greece for more than 22 weeks of gestation. Moreover, the implementation of treatment programs for pregnant women with symptoms of threatened preterm delivery, failed to reduce the incidence of preterm birth [12–14]. The lack of progress may be partly related to the increase in the frequency of multiple pregnancies as a result of the widespread use of assisted reproduction methods, but the main cause remains largely unclear. The incidence of prematurity (23rd-24th weeks to <37 weeks) in the US, for single pregnancies is 9.43%, for twins 50.74% and for triplets 91.03%.

It has also been observed that opposed to the Caucasian race, the black race is associated with an increased rate of low birth weight neonates and preterm delivery. There is great heterogeneity within the same racial group, however members of the same race may have different frequency of precocities in different geographical areas. The differences remain even after the control for the social order. The racial difference has not decreased over time. The mother's race is a stronger indicator of precocity than the father's race, although the father's race is also important. The probability that the racial difference is genetically determined is based on data showing different distribution of gestational age in the black and white population. The gestational age distributions for black and non-black women appear to deviate by 1 week, resulting in a mean gestational age of 39 weeks for blacks 37 and 40 weeks for whites [15–20].

Approximately 1/3 of health expenditures in infancy and childhood are due to complications of preterm delivery as 10% of surviving infants have long-term disabilities such as developmental or behavioral problems [12–14]. The Financial Cost in US for health care amounts to 9 billion $/year and the 35% of the expenses is for newborns and 10% for children. Also, the high cost of hospitalization of newborns <1500 g should be emphasized in intensive care units [12–14]. In Germany, out of a total of 50,000 preterm births (BP) and the annual cost are as follows: PB <32 weeks 300 million €, PB ≥ 32 weeks 400 million € and cost for tocolysis 112 million €.

It is estimated that about 85% of neonatal deaths in Western countries are attributed to prematurity and 10% of these neonates will suffer from some form of long-term disability. Of the reported rate of prematurity, 10% of the neonates delivered before the 37th week of pregnancy, about 1.5% before the end of the 32nd week and approximately 0.5% of premature births will take place in the period before the 28th week [12–14]. Premature birth is a potentially very serious problem for newborns and the morbidity and mortality rates are inversely proportional to the maturity of the organic systems, especially the lungs [6, 21].

In particular, in the 22nd week of pregnancy, the temporary survival rate is 40%, respiratory distress syndrome 70%, intra-abdominal bleeding 25%, sepsis 25% and necrotic enterocolitis 8% with a final survival rate of 5% [6, 21]. Some of the following changes are observed between 22nd and 34th week of pregnancy: sepsis 4%, increase of temporary survival to 97% reduction of respiratory distress syndrome to 14%, intra-abdominal bleeding 0%, necrotic 3% with intestinal necrosis final survival 97% [6–11]. The prognosis of newborns improves when the gestation period is prolonged. Recent literature reports indicate the following neonatal survival rates: at 23 weeks 6–9%, at 24 weeks 17–58%, at 25 weeks 35–85%, at 27–28 weeks 90% and at 33 weeks 95%.

3. Risk factors of preterm birth stimulation

Primary risk factors:

- Multiple pregnancies
- History of preterm birth
- History of threatened preterm birth
- Abdominal surgery during pregnancy

- Congenital uterine abnormalities
- History of automatic miscarriages
- History of conical resection
- Cervical removal> 30%
- Polyamnium
- Presence of intense myometrial activity
- Cervical dilation> 2 cm

Secondary risk factors:

- Feverish disease in pregnancy
- Bleeding in the 2nd trimester
- History of acute pyelonephritis
- History of miscarriage in the 2nd trimester
- Smoking more than 10 cigarettes per day

4. Maternal causes and conditions in pregnancy related to preterm birth

4.1 Socio-economic and racial factors

The low socio-economic status of pregnant women related to education, employment or family income and racial, demographic, environmental factors is one of the most common factors associated with the occurrence of preterm birth. Statistically, a causal relationship has been found between the economic situation and the low level of education.

Mothers with a low level of education are more likely to give birth to low birth weight babies and less likely to give birth to large babies. The average birth weight increases with the greater education of the mother. White mothers with 12 years of education, on average, had 82 g heavier babies than mothers with less education, while the corresponding difference for newborns born to black women was 66 g. Mothers with ≥12 years of education had even heavier neonates. The risk of having a very low birth weight neonate has been shown to vary depending on the level of education among white, but not among black women [11, 22–26].

Newborns born from low-educated mothers are less likely to survive. Low-educated mothers have characteristics that are blamed for the birth of low birth weight babies. They are more likely to be young, have less prenatal care, smoke during pregnancy, have a poor diet and have more difficult access to medical care. Also, women in lower social classes have higher levels of stress with elevated catecholamine levels that can lead to increased uterine contractions. Better education of the mother could improve her diet, reduce smoking during pregnancy but also reduce other harmful factors [11, 22–26].

4.2 Maternal age

Maternal age (under 19 or over 35) is associated with an increased incidence of preterm birth [27–30]. However, the risk may not come from age itself but from the factors associated with it. For the young women, it is more usual to suffering of vaginitis than the older women, which may have other health problems, such as fibroids, hypertension and metabolic diseases [15–20]. Also, women with body weight before pregnancy under 50 kg and height below 150 cm, have higher rates of preterm birth. Therefore, chronological age is not an independent factor of gestational age but the increased risks reflect characteristics of the mother's advanced age.

Great importance was given to the premature birth of women over 35 years old due to the growing population of pregnant women with first pregnancies at an older age. However, there are views on the increased risk in those over the age of 30, compared to women aged 20–29. Maybe due to the improvement of perinatal care, the relative risk of preterm delivery in women aged >35 years old, decreased from 1.7% in 1976 to 1% in 1981. Adolescent white women give birth to newborns that are lighter by 149gr, while black women by 99gr, compared to those of mothers aged 20–34 years. Mothers aged 35 years and older give birth to children which are 50gr heavier than those of women 20–34 years [15–20].

Neonatal mortality is also slightly higher in younger and older women.

4.3 Burdened obstetric history

The existence of a burdened obstetric history seems to be directly related to the frequency of preterm birth. Miscarriages, especially in the second trimester, previous preterm births and stillbirths, increase the risk of premature births in subsequent pregnancies. A previous history of low birth weight or preterm birth is one of the most important factors for the next preterm birth. The literature states that the relative risk with a history of preterm birth is 34%, while it is even higher for the third childbirth, although both previous ones were premature. Racial differences have been observed in the relationship between first and second preterm birth, while the previous history of preterm birth is a significant risk factor for premature rupture of membranes.

The number of pregnancies does not seem to affect the likelihood of preterm birth as the results of several studies are contradictory. It is generally accepted that first-born infants weigh less on average compared to their offspring at each gestational age. The explanation for the reported data is not known. It is possible that fetal development is more limited in primiparous pregnant women, due to the anatomy of the muscular walls of the uterus, compared to those with multiple pregnancies [15–20].

There is an increased risk of preterm birth compared to the short interval between two pregnancies, but the results are not statistically significant. It is therefore not clear whether there is any relationship between short interval between births and prematurity.

4.4 Previous stillbirths or neonatal deaths

4.4.1 Previous induced abortions

The contribution of abortions to the increased risk of premature birth depends on the type of abortion, the degree of dilation of the cervix, the gestational age and the number of abortions [15–20].

4.4.2 History of infertility

Women who have undergone assisted reproduction therapy in single pregnancies show a prematurity rate of 10–20%. The increase is due to pre-existing reproductive abnormalities, an increased rate of multiple pregnancies, and an increasing number of cesarean sections before the 37th week of pregnancy.

4.5 Various diseases of the mother

Maternal diseases related to pregnancy (e.g. preeclampsia and eclampsia) or unrelated to pregnancy (chronic kidney disease, anemia, chronic hypertension, respiratory failure, etc.) are common causes of premature birth or low birth weight babies. Most of these diseases cause pathology in the placental circulation resulting in problematic fetal development and low body weight. Also the most well-known of the endocrine diseases associated with increased prematurity are diabetes mellitus and hyperthyroidism [20, 31–35].

4.5.1 Smoking and alcohol

Smoking seems to be responsible for an increased rate of prematurity, is associated with placental abruption and perinatal mortality. This effect of smoking is attributed to the increase in anthracylamoglobin and the action of nicotine. Also various toxins also known as Cyanide reduce the levels of vitamin B12 resulting in metabolic disorders. Anthracycline hemoglobin increases from 1.2% to 4.1% and reduces the oxygen available for fetal oxygenation while nicotine increases epinephrine secretion and causes vasoconstriction, further aggravating fetal oxygenation [20, 31–35].

Alcohol abuse, in addition to its association with prematurity, has also been linked to an increased risk of brain damage in premature infants.

4.5.2 Illegal drug use

Marijuana and cocaine have been studied more for their potential effects on preterm birth. There is no serious evidence that marijuana is associated with prematurity. In contrast, cocaine has been studied much more with a wealth of literature linking its use to preterm birth [20, 31–35].

4.5.3 Medical monitoring

Inadequate medical follow-up, as expressed by the late first visit of the pregnant woman and the limited number of visits, has a direct impact on the increase of prematurity. This is confirmed by the increased rate of prematurity in pregnant women, especially in adolescent pregnant women who are not monitored by their personal doctor or midwife, where the system of free medical care applies [20, 31–35].

4.5.4 Surgical diseases during pregnancy

Acute surgical diseases of the abdomen, such as acute appendicitis, are associated with an increased incidence of preterm birth due to the effect of bacterial endotoxins [20, 31–35].

4.5.5 Uterine congenital abnormalities and diseases

Uterine congenital abnormalities characterized as anatomical are responsible for a small percentage of preterm births. The most common occurrences are in the double uterus, unicorn, duodenum and hypoplastic uterus where the incidence of miscarriage is close to 30% and the risk of premature birth reaches 20% if the pregnancy continues beyond the 20th week of pregnancy. There is also an association with prematurity and fibroids, endometrial adhesions idiopathic myometrial activity [20, 31–35].

4.5.6 *Insufficiency of internal cervical os*

The uterus and cervix come from the union of M*ü*ller ducts. The cervix is made up of extracellular connective tissue and type I, III and IV collagen fibers. The percentage of smooth muscle fibers is 10–15%. The percentage of muscle and fibrous components ranges from 29% in the inner cervix to 6% in the outer cervix. Other components of the cervix are glycosaminoglycans, proteoglycans, fibronectin and elastin. Before and during labour, the number of ligaments between the collagen fibers decreases, the concentration of hyaluronic acid increases and this leads to elimination and dilation of the cervix and uterine contractions.

Internal cervical insufficiency is a fairly common cause of prematurity. Also a history with conical resection of the cervix is responsible for an increased rate of premature birth which is observed with a frequency of 14% for the first pregnancy and quadruples in subsequent ones [35–40].

4.5.7 *Maternal infections*

Inflammations of the vagina and cervix caused by anaerobic microbes, Trichomonas, Chlamydia, gonococci and streptococci of group B, usually lead to premature birth, premature rupture of membranes and low birth weight infants. With preventive examinations at the beginning of pregnancy such as vaginal fluid culture and the application of treatment in case of positive results, we achieve the reduction of the possibility for premature birth [35–40].

Subclinical chorioamnionitis can predispose to preterm birth. However, the infection is associated with less than 20% of cases of premature birth without complications. The most common link between infection and premature birth is bacterial vaginosis. Disruption of the nitric acid and prostaglandin balance of the myometrium can cause premature contractions and consequent labor.

The vagina is normally colonized by a variety of microorganisms, many of which are flora, while others are potentially pathogenic. It is not fully known whether the bacterial flora itself acts as a trigger for preterm birth or secondarily becomes active only when the cervix is unable to fulfill its protection against incurable infections. Ascending infection is one of the most important mechanisms that progress to premature birth. The infection can act as a trigger, either in the sense that it is more likely to lead to premature birth when the cervix is open at the end of pregnancy, or when the cervix opens prematurely. The degree of cervical dilation affects the risk of ascending infection.

Infection that occurs with intact embryonic membranes reduces infection by the flora of the vagina and cervix. The incidence of amniotic fluid infection varies depending on gestational age at birth. It is particularly high in very premature fetuses and gradually decreases at 30–34 weeks and remains stable until the end of pregnancy [35–40].

4.5.8 *Infection of the lower urinary tract*

The essential role of the infection in preterm birth was confirmed by the finding in the amniotic fluid or the dermis and the amniotic fluid of women with pathogenic microorganisms (Ureoplasma urealiticun, Mycoplasma hominis, *Streptococcus agalactiae*). In particular, the detection rate of the above infectious microorganisms during pregnancy according to the literature is Ureoplasma urealiticun 60%, Trichomonas vaginalis 34%, Mycoplasma hominis20%, Streptococcus agalacticae 5–18% and Gardanerella vaginallis 12% anerobe. Chorioamniosis colonization was twice as much as amniotic fluid. This colonization was more common and inversely proportional to the gestational age and birth weight of the newborn, in women with intact membranes whose labor was spontaneous, compared with women of the same gestational age who gave birth due to medical or obstetric indications other than automatic childbirth. The inverse relationship between positive choriamnia cultures and gestational age was not observed in women giving birth due to medical indications [35–40].

Among women who gave birth up to 30 weeks by spontaneous delivery, choriamnius culture was positive in 73%, compared with 21% of births due to indications. Horiamnius cultures were positive in 83% of mothers with spontaneous onset of labor and in 16% of mothers who gave birth due to indications, in newborns weighing less than 1000 g. An equal number of newborns are born at gestational ages who have proinflammatory cytokines in the amniotic fluid, with negative fluid culture, so that the majority of newborns born under 26 weeks and a significant proportion of those born under 30 weeks have inflammation or inflammation amniotic fluid These findings are mirrored in histological studies of the dermis and amniotic fluid, infiltrated by polymorphonuclear neutrophils in almost all pregnancies of 20–23 weeks, in the majority of those under 26 weeks, and in a significant proportion of those born before 30 weeks [35–40].

The reason for the high frequency of infections - inflammations in the amniotic fluid and chorioamnion is inexplicable in very premature pregnancies under 26 weeks, even under 30 weeks. The flora studies are incomplete from the beginning to the 23rd week of pregnancy, while from the 23rd to the end they show a rather stable vaginal flora [35–40].

The cervix begins to change composition and have maturation elements between 20 and 26 weeks, under the influence of biochemical changes (prostaglandins and interleukin) and uterine contractions. Changes in the cervix increase the exposure to vaginal cervical bacteria of the upper cervix, lower uterus and chorioamnion, resulting in increased amniotic fluid and chorioamnion infection, the most vulnerable barrier between the fetus and the environment.

Most amniotic infections are subclinical, with no maternal fever, uterine tenderness, tachycardia, or foul-smelling amniotic fluid. Very often, however, the mother's infection is not obvious until the infection of the fetus begins. The only fetal sign indicative of amniotic infection is fetal tachycardia, an unstable symptom of systemic neonatal infection. But what makes an amniotic infection fetal and not maternal? The fetus first responds to the infection by responding to the fetal part of the chorioamnion. Proinflammatory cytokines and prostaglandins accumulate in the amniotic fluid. A systemic fetal immune response occurs and produces proinflammatory cytokines and other evidence in the fetal blood [35–40].

Periodontitis has also been studied in women who have low birth weight neonates, resulting from either spontaneous preterm delivery or premature rupture of membranes. It has been found that these mothers have more severe periodontal disease than those who give birth to normal weight babies. It is possible that oral infection with Gram (−) anaerobic microbes fusobacterium nucleutatum, to act periodically, as a chronic factor of hematogenous dispersion of bacteria or bacterial agents (lipopolysaccharides and endotoxins), in the placental unit [35–40].

5. Causes and conditions of embryoplacutic unit related to preterm birth

5.1 Multiple pregnancies

A multiple pregnancy is at greater risk for preterm birth due to the continuous dilation of the uterus and the onset of premature contractions. If the average pregnancy is 280.5 days, in twin pregnancies it is 261 days and in triplets is 247 days [41–44].

5.2 Congenital fetal abnormalities

Increased rate of prematurity due to uterine overstretching is due to polyamine and especially hydramnios. The 1/3 of pregnancies with polyamnios leads to premature birth. The main causes of polyamniosis are congenital abnormalities of the fetus's nervous and digestive systems, intestinal obstruction, septal hernia, Potter's like Syndrome, Skeletal Deformities (Amniotic bands <24 weeks), chromosomal abnormalities, infections. In particular, hydramnios is associated with congenital abnormalities of the fetal nervous system such as aneurysm (due to polydramnios), renal agenesis (due to oligamnius) in combination with pulmonary hypoplasia and endogenous metabolic disorders and some of them are causative factors of preterm birth [45–50].

5.3 Abnormalities of the placenta and umbilicus

Abnormalities in the morphology, implantation and function of the placenta can often lead to premature birth. Placentas with membranous umbilical cord protrusion are at greater risk for premature onset of labor. Also the precursor placenta is an important factor in causing premature birth. It is characteristic that it is more common in premature births than in normal ones. Premature placental abruption has an even higher incidence in preterm birth than in normal.

5.4 Breech fetal presentation

Breech presentation of the fetus in the first trimester of pregnancy has an incidence of 20% compared to all pregnancies and only 2% of this percentage leads to premature birth. However, sciatic projection is associated with increased perinatal mortality as well as placental abnormalities thus increasing the likelihood of preterm delivery.

5.5 Premature rupture of membranes

Spontaneous rupture of fetal membranes (s-PROM) before the end of 37 weeks and 1 hour before the onset of labor covers 14.3% in all preterm births. It is distinguished in term Premature Rupture of membranes (t-PROM) which is defined as rupture of membranes after the 37th week of pregnancy and constitutes the majority of cases and in preterm Premature rupture of membranes (p-PROM) which is defined as rupture of membranes before the 37th week of pregnancy has an incidence of 3% and is responsible for 40% of preterm births. Its incidence is 10–15% of pregnancies.

Findings observed are contractions (4 per 20 min or 8 per 60 min) and cervical dilation >2 cm and/or cervical effacement >80%. It is associated with complications related to the outcome of pregnancy and perinatal outcome, increases the chance of premature birth and neonatal morbidity and mortality to 1–2% [45–50].

The incidence rates are 6% - 10% <37 weeks, 1.5% <32 weeks, 0.5% <28 weeks. Often there is no obvious predisposing factor. The main causes of PROM are malnutrition, vaginitis, cervical insufficiency, abnormalities of the uterus. Pregnancy usually precedes the same episode. The diagnosis of PROM is based on the history of the pregnant woman where discharge from the vagina is reported. The differential diagnosis from other conditions (alkaline urine, inflammation) is usually made by direct examination of the cervical spine and by testing the sunflower map.

The complications of PROM, in addition to those of prematurity, include inflammation of the mother and the fetal placenta, as well as umbilical cord prolapse, which implies significant perinatal morbidity and mortality [45–50]. Babies born with symptoms of sepsis are 4 times more likely to have neonatal mortality than those who do not. In addition, there are risks for the mother from the complications of possible chorioamnionitis [45–50].

Diagnosis is not always easy. It seems that taking a good medical history and then examining the woman using a vaginal dilator helps a lot. Moreover, obstetric ultrasound is helpful in diagnosis. Specifically, the presence of amniotic fluid in the posterior vaginal dome is very helpful in the diagnosis. The nitrazine test and the microscopic examination of the amniotic fluid for the typical image of the fern, have a sensitivity of 90% with false positives of 17% and 6%, respectively due to the mixture of urine and blood or cervical mucus, respectively.

6. PROM monitoring

Criteria for diagnosing chorioamnionitis include: fever, tachycardia, fetal tachycardia, odorous vaginal fluids, leukocytosis and uterine tenderness. Vitals are taken every 4–8 hours and the existence of one or a combination of the above findings raises the suspicion of fetal infection. Doppler ultrasound, biophysical profile and fetal heart rate have been used from time to time in various studies to distinguish infected fetuses from non-infected ones and therefore pregnancy can be prolonged without success in distinguishing which fetuses are in risk and which not.

Women should be monitored clinically for signs of chorioamnionitis. Apart from vaginal fluid culture at the time of introduction no other need to be taken on a weekly basis. According to the American College of Obstetricians and Gynecologists, CRP and white blood cell count should be checked twice a week. No daily blood draws are needed for leukocytosis and CRP, due to the low sensitivity. Biophysical and Doppler can be done but have no significant prognostic value [45–50].

6.1 Role of antibiotics

Although different regimens have been used in various studies (penicillins, erythromycin, clindamycin, from 2 doses - 10 days) it seems that the prolongation of pregnancy is stable and the morbidity for mother and newborn is reduced. It is recommended 5–7 days administration of macrolides (erythromycin, azithromycin). Clindamycin is preferred when there is allergy in the first option.

Administration of ceftriaxone, clarithromycin metronidazole β-lactam, appears to significantly extend the time to delivery and the frequency of chorioamnionitis (23 vs. 12 days, p: 0.01, and 50% vs. 67%, p: 0.05, respectively). Finally, there are insufficient data to prove the direct favorable contribution of antibiotics in reducing neonatal morbidity and mortality. Nevertheless the combination of the mentioned antibiotics used as empirical therapy against the aforementioned germs ureaplasma, mycoplasma, anaerobes and gram negative bacteria according to bibliographic data offered satisfactory results in the early and early rupture of fetal membranes for both the mother and the fetus. Strategy for treating a subclinical possible infection. The administration of clavulanic acid should be avoided due to the possible cause of necrotic enterocolitis in the fetus and in cases of group B streptococci additional antibiotics should be given during delivery. Antibiotics are effective in treating infection without being able to prevent a premature birth.

6.2 Role of steroids

According to the instructions of the American College of Obstetricians and Gynecologists, it is recommended to administer a single dose of steroids in pregnancies <32 weeks with PPROM that do not show signs of infection. Two meta-analyzes conclude that steroids in PPROM significantly reduce Respiratory Difficulty Syndrome, encephalopathy and intra-abdominal bleeding. It does not appear to increase the rate of infection from their administration. A single dose should be given to pregnant women from 24 to 34 weeks. The manifolds are associated with a smaller head size and smaller birth weight [45–50].

6.3 Role of tocolysis

Tocolysis in women with CPR is not recommended because this treatment does not statistically significantly improve perinatal outcome. The administration of tocolysis to women with CPR and contractions to act on steroids and antibiotics remains unclear. Attempting to suppress preterm uterine-related contractions using first-line tocolytic therapy can achieve prolongation of gestational age. Among the administered tocolytics, β-sympathomimetics do not excel in the other categories in terms of their effectiveness and in addition are associated with a negligible rate of side effects. Conservative treatment with β-sympathomimetics or magnesium offers almost nothing in the whole treatment effort. Careful selection of cases is recommended. Hospitalization for 48–72 hours may be needed, but other than that, informing pregnant woman about possible symptoms of chorioamnionitis is necessary (e.g. temperature measurement).

6.4 PROM and cerclage

There are no randomized studies on what should be done in such cases. Some studies show a tendency for chorioamnionitis to start earlier, while others show a prolongation of pregnancy. The risks and benefits of suturing for a short time until steroids work have not been adequately studied [45–50].

6.5 PROM and childbirth

Childbirth should be scheduled between 34th and 40th weeks. If extended beyond this time limit the pregnant woman should be explained the increased chance of choriamnionitis and the reduced chance of respiratory problems from the newborn. In Premature Childbirth the hypoxia is greater compared to that of a full term. Vaginal delivery is recommended at a young gestational age (≤ 25th week). In fetal difficulty many suggest cesarean section. Between 26th and 34th week is no different from the way after 34th week. Vaginal childbirth is the appropriate route of completion of childbirth when there are no abnormal shapes and projections, elements of fetal difficulty, e.g. IUGR [45–50].

Iatrogenic PROM occurs after deliberate medical intervention, when it is estimated that continued pregnancy is at greater risk for the mother and fetus than prematurity.

Complications of the placenta: placental abruption, placenta previa.

Amniotic fluid complications: oligamnium, polyamnion, chorioamnionitis, premature rupture of membranes.

Fetal causes: congenital anomalies, multiple pregnancy, residual development, fetal discomfort.

7. Pathophysiology of preterm labor

Activation of the maternal/fetal hypothalamic–pituitary–adrenal axis (HPA) due to maternal or fetal stress: connection between maternal psychosocial stress and preterm birth - mechanism similar to normal childbirth.

The following factors such as: Stress, Autoimmune mechanisms, PROM, Inflammation, Bleeding, Uterine overdistension, Multiple pregnancies, disorders of axis (pituitary axis), Inflammation, Environmental factors, Social factors, Activation of mechanisms, induction of contractions leading to effacement and dilation of cervix and finally labor [51–56].

Chorioamnionitis or systemic inflammation from systemic or ascending infection: cervical, decidual and fetal membrane's cytokines activation (macrophage activation, production of interleukins IL 1, IL 6, IL 8, cachectin, 5-hydroxytryptheptamine, release of fibronectin in cervical and vaginal secretions).

Bleeding from decidual: three or seven fold risk of prematurity, especially as a result of premature rupture of membranes.

Uterine oversdistension: myometrial stimulation, increased cytokine expression [50–60].

7.1 Preterm labor: the mechanism includes

Activation of the maternal and/or fetal HPA axis (psychological or physical stress).

Inflammatory reaction - local or systemic.

Bleeding from decidual.

Increased uterine stretching (multiple pregnancies, hydramnion).

Cervical insufficiency.

Activation of HPA axis.

An increase of CRH levels (corticosteroids) can cause a raise of PG (Prostaglandin) levels and consequently an increase of the MMPs (metalloproteinases) activity, Activation of metals of protein (MMPs) of the parent substance (MMP-1, −3, −8, −9) leads to degradation of the fibrous tissue, and premature rupture of membranes. Bacterial products and/or profibrous cytokines acting on cervical cells of the uterus may cause a change of MMPs expression. High concentrations MMP-8 of amniotic fluid are associated with PB (before the 32nd week of pregnancy) so induction of uterine contractions (directly or by functional "withdrawal" of progesterone) [50–60].

The angiogenic factor VEGF, expressed in embryonic membranes and perishable, is essentially involved in normal angiogenesis and placentalization - thus ensuring way to normal fetal growth and development - while at the same time modifying its permeability in placenta and amniotic membranes. Daneshmand et al. and Kramer et al. suggest that both the VEGF factor and (VEGF-R1 and VEGF-R2) receptors have reduced expression in hypoxic conditions and chorioamnionitis, disrupt the smooth functioning of placental abruption and lead to PB. Similarly, Parazoglou et al. proved the correlation among two common VEGF functional gene polymorphisms (−634G/C and 936C/T) with PB [50–60].

In case of preterm labor, CRH levels are ≥ 2 MoM.

Elevated levels of ACTH (Cortical Adrenal Hormone) and CRH can result in raised levels of DHEA (dehydroepiandrosterone) and 16-OH-DHEA-S (dehydroepiandrosterone sulfate) as increased E1 (estrone) – E3 (estradiole). As a result uterine contractions are induced. (Activation through binding in oxytocin receptors, involvement of MLCK (myosin light chain kinase) and calmodulin. Increased E3 in saline is observed in premature labor, 3–4 weeks before delivery.

Inflammatory reaction is mediated through the following cytokine agents:

Cytokines, TNF-α, Il-1, Il-1β, Il-6, Il-8, Il-10, GM-CSF and finally prostagladines increase.

Fetal membranes, trophoblast and the chorionic villi react, in response to inflammation and ischemic lesions of placental unit and cause an increase in cytokines levels in maternal plasma, in the amniotic fluid of women with preterm labor and in cultures of amniotic fluid.

TNF-α is also found in decidual macrophages as well as in chorion villi and trophoblast. The TNF-α factor is found in maperishable cells of perishables, villi and trophoblast, in both the 1st and 3rd trimester of pregnancy. Its allele gene A region −308 of the TNF-α promoter leads to an increase production of it. Roberts et al. reported positive correlation between polymorphism of the TNF-α promoter region (−308 A allele) and the PB and/or premature rupture among African American women [50–60].

On the contrary, Amory et al. found that homozygotes for the TNF-α allele-863 A gene is significantly increased frequency of PB, chorionicamniotnitis and perinatal morbidity, but this is not associated with an adverse outcome. Il-1 is detected in amniotic fluid, in decidua and trophoblast. The receptor antagonist of IL-1 inhibits the biological effects of IL-1, blocking its receptors. Consequently reduction of IL-1 production and induced from that of prostaglandin production by them endometrial tissue can prevent PB associated with infection Il-1β is found in chorionic villi, decidua, amniotic fluid and placental cultures [50–60]. Elevated levels of Il-6 are usually found in the amniotic fluid, with inflammation. Interleukin-6 (IL-6) is the cytokine expressed more than any other in pregnancy. The finding of extremelly high levels of the specific cytokine in the amniotic fluid pregnant women who presented with some kind of inflammation and its very low concentration in cases of PB "idiopathic" etiology, make it one of the most sensitive and specific PB indicators On the contrary, they were found to be reduced in cases of premature birth. Il-10 is also elevated in amniotic fluid after amniocentesis during the second trimester in pregnancies with IUGR and chorioamnionitis [50–60]. Interleukin-10 (IL-10) is known to be major inhibitory cytokine in the process synthesis of cytokines by both T cells (interferon-γ and IL-2), as well as by monocytes macrophages (TNF-α, IL-6, IL-8, and IL-12) and as therefore plays an important role in achieving the outcome of the pregnancy by securing the maternity tolerance to the allogeneic fetus. In most pregnancies IL-10 is detected in amniotic fluid Its high levels in amniotic fluid of pregnancies complicated with residual embryonic development as well as in cases of pregnant women with clinical symptoms chorioamnionitis associated with dysfunctional for immune activity in pregnancy and in PB [50–60].

Increased levels of interleukin-8 (IL-8) are found in monocytes, in inflammation, in chorioamnionitis and may be used in the future as a prognostic marker of preterm birth. Interleukin-8 (IL-8), a derivative of monocytes; caused by inflammation, may be used in the future as a PB predictor marker as it has been detected in pregnant women.

Inter twined with chorioamnionitis, and the antigen compatibility (also a derivative of macrocells, which is considered necessary in cellular immune response) is associated with inflammation of the elements of pregnancy.

Bacteria, specially their wall lipoproteins and/or endotoxins can stimulate an increase of IL-1β, TNF-α, IL-8, IL-6, proteases, collagenase, elastase as well as raise of Phospholipase A2 led to PGF2a endothelins and finally increase the myometrial sensitivity to oxytocin [51–56].

7.2 Chorioamnionitis

It is observed in 12% of premature labors with intact membranes. Histological diagnosis of chorioamnionitis is 40% confirmed in the placenta.

It is also known that frequency of choriomnionitis is inversely proportional with gestational age.

8. Preterm labor and genetic background

8.1 Modern molecular biology certifies a premature gene

Quickly developing fields studying human genome (genomic) and protein products (proteomic) may allow the identification of genes and proteins respectively involved in the pathology of PT, making in this way it is possible to develop concrete diagnostic and therapeutic approaches against that. The use of DNA arrays helps to identify the different gene expression and their involvement in childbirth, early or full term.

Reduced expression insulin-dependent factor II (IGF-II), of galgranulin A and B (calgranulin A and B) and of the G-protein-binding receptor (G-protein-coupled receptor) was observed in the myometrium during childbirth - in contrast increased expression of the binding genes protein storage of insulin-dependent IGFs (IGF-binding protein), the binding of the Ca2+/CaM ion protein (Ca2+/CaM binding protein), the C-kinase substrate (kinase C substrate) and the converting enzyme of angiotensin-converting enzyme is noticed. Also, the use of DNA arrays in expression of their cytokine genes fetal membranes of women with endometrial inflammation and who gave birth prematurely, showed hyper-expression in 22 genes and sub-expression in 4 on a total of 90 of genes studied. The IL-1β genes of oncostatin M and the enhancer pre-B-cell enhancing factor factor) were those with the greatest difference expression.

These studies demonstrate the potential for genomic research in the identification of genes involved in the pathophysiology of complex diseases, as in the case of PB.

Although the results of studies with the use DNA arrays may show significant over- or under-expression in a set of genes, that not necessarily related to level changes of their protein expression [50–60].

DNA analysis is based on molecular biology methods, such as:

1. The investigation of the functional variability of the candidate gene.

2. Northern blots analysis.

3. Linkage analysis.

4. Subtractive hybridization.

Mutations and polymorphisms in the cytokine genes seem to be involved in pathogenesis of preterm labor. There is an association between preterm labor and the functional change of a cytokine gene. So, mother's carriers of this mutations, may be can be intensively followed up in the future [51–56].

Proteolytic action of MMPs on fetal membranes and cervical mucus leads to progressive cervical effacement and therefore to PROM.

Bleeding observed in more than 2 trimesters increases the relative risk of PROM 7 times.

According to Salafia et al. [61], in 38% of preterm labors hematoma and/or hemosiderin deposition was detected, instead 0.8% in full-term pregnancies.

According to Gargano et al. [62], in cases of preterm labor, Factor V Leyden & angiotensinogen -6G mutations are associated with an increased relative risk (OR: 4.8) of placental abruption in Caucasians but not in African-American pregnant women.

It is also found increased frequency of PROM in women with increased TF (tissue factor - major cellular mediator of hemostasis).

Uterine overdistension due to multiple pregnancy or polydydramnios are the most common risk factors for preterm labor. Uterine distension leads to oxytocin receptors activation and increase of PG and MLCK.

According to Nemeth et al. [63] fetal membranes rupture stimulate the cytokines, PGs and collagenase production. Warren et al. [64] suggest that cervical incompetence may have a genetic background alleles that control anti-inflammatory mediators, that were found in women with high risk for cervical incompetence. Sanbhag et al. [65] women diagnosed with CIN III are in high risk for preterm labor even have not been cured by cone-biopsy. Congenital cervical incompetence is basically rare [51–56].

In conclusion, preterm labor seems to be a result of the following mechanisms:

1. Factors stimulated the HPA axon activation.

2. Inflammatory response.

3. Decidual bleeding.

4. Uterine overdistension.

Common mechanism– Contraction associated proteins (CAPs) and proteases production.

9. Preterm labor prediction

To predict preterm labor are suggested:

1. Cervical ultrasound evaluation (18–24 Weeks).

   Combination of cervical length and funneling significantly increases the possibility of preterm labor.
   Combination of cervical length and dilatation of internal os, increases the sensitivity, but only 29%.

2. Fetal fibronectin (FFN).

10. Recommendation as routine method in high risk pregnancies

Nowadays, diagnostic view is focused on score systems that combine ultrasound, biochemical and endocrinologic parameters with molecular methods, such as fetal DNA measurement in maternal circulation. Not rarely, among asymptomatic or low risk pregnancies may be can be found high risk pregnancies for preterm labor.

There is a significant statistical correlation between preterm labor and cervical length <20 mm–25 mm [56, 66–69].

11. Controversial aspects for the efficacy of ultrasound examination

Transvaginal cervical length measurement between 18 and 24 weeks is commonly suggested as a reliable index of preterm labor. On the other hand, some studies support that generalized preventive cervical measurement has no sufficient evidence.

The timing of cervical measurement in asymptomatic pregnancies with increased risk for preterm labor (history of preterm labor and history of PROM) seems to significantly affect the estimated risk of preterm labor.

Some other studies propose the combination of cervical length measurement and the detection of fetal fibronectin.

Transvaginal ultrasound confirm the preterm labor diagnosis in high risk pregnancies, especially when was applied in the first trimester.

Regarding the cervical cerclage as a method of preventing preterm labor, we clearly suggest that it should be performed only in women with previous history of preterm labor and if ultrasound examinations indicate cervical incompetence.

12. Biochemical markers of preterm labor

1. Vaginocervical cytokines

2. Vaginocervical and/or proteases

3. Maternal and/or fetal distress index CRH (Corticotropin-releasing hormone) estradiol, estriol (plasma, urine)

4. Fibronectin (vaginocervical)

12.1 Vaginocervical fetal fibronectin (fFN)

Vaginocervical fetal fibronectin (fFN) is a glycoprotein of the extracellular matrix that affects the maintenance of placental adherence to the maternal decidua. Generally, fFN can be found in cervicovaginal fluid early in gestation until 20th week. The detection of fFN after the 20 week may indicate a disruption of the decidual-chorionic interface of the amniotic membrane and is linked with a significant increased risk of preterm labor. Diagnostic tests based on fFN have sensitivity 81.7% and specificity 82.5%.

The absence of FFN is a strong marker that preterm labor is unlikely to occur within the next 7–14 days. So, negative prognostic value in some studies exceeding 99%. The prognostic value of FFN is higher in pregnancies 24–28 weeks, in comparison with older gestational ages and much stronger for short-term predictions (7–14 days), than in using for the overall outcome [56, 66–69].

13. Preterm labor diagnosis

Painful contractions are observed at regular intervals combined with progressive effacement and dilation of the cervix. However in 50% of cases contractions may not induce premature labor.

14. Pre-symptomatic control for preterm labor

Cervical assessment is necessary to evaluate the risk for preterm labor. Cervical length <15 mm observed in 2% of women in 23th w, in 90% of cases happens labor before 28 weeks.

Cervical length >15 mm implies 4% risk for preterm labor.

Cervical length < 5 mm implies 78% risk for preterm labor.

High Bishop's score increases the risk of preterm labor.

Using the ultrasound cervical length measurement we have to remember that normal average is about 34–40 mm, without bulging of the fetal membranes into the internal os. The major risk factor coming from obstetric history that can be used for the evaluation of preterm risk in the current pregnancy is the previous preterm labor. Avoiding factors as urinary tract infections, vaginal infections, smoking, drug abuse and physically demanding work is also important [56, 66–73].

14.1 Fetal fibronectin measurement

Fetal fibronectin helps to maintain the integrity of the extracellular matrix between chorion villi and basal decidua. It is usually not detected after 20 weeks and until the membranes rupture happens.

If fibronectin was detected, the risk of preterm labor significantly increases.

The presence of fibronectin at 23 weeks implies 60% possibility for labor before 28th week.

15. Preterm neonates and prematurity complications

The prematurity importance is related to the complications that brings both for the newborn survival as well as for the later development. These complications are often unknown and maybe have unclear long-term effects. Medical decisions are normally defined by the possible effects in combination with the available information depending on the gestational age.

Complications of preterm labor arise from immature systems and organs that are not able to normally function in a ecto-uterine environment. The risk of acute neonatal disease decreases with advancing gestational age demonstrating the fragility of the brain, lungs, immune system, kidneys, skin, eyes and gastrointestinal tract.

15.1 Disorders of preterm neonates

The following are the most important acute and chronic problems faced by premature infants admitted to the Intensive Care Unit. More specifically, these refer the developmental and mental retardation, cerebral palsy, deafness, blindness, transient dystonia, feeding difficulties and speech delay [70–83].

15.1.1 Disorders of thermoregulation

Premature infants usually present difficulties in thermoregulation due to the immaturity of the homeostatic mechanism of production and elimination. Contributing factors include the large ratio of body surface area/weight, thin and immature skin, immaturity of the autonomic nervous system and incomplete development of sweat glands that can allow increased heat and fluid loss.

15.1.2 Newborn respiratory distress syndrome

Newborn Respiratory Distress Syndrome (NRBS) or hyaline membrane disease is caused due to the deficiency of surfactant factor and is clinically manifested with respiratory distress of varying severity. Its frequency is inversely proportional to gestational age, reaching 80% for premature infants born before 28 weeks. Surfactant factor is produced by pneumocytes type II and reduces cell surface tension by preventing the development of atelectasis at the end of expiration.

In premature infants, in which the surfactant is deficient, cell atelectasis develops and gas exchange is disrupted. Newborns with RDS show respiratory distress immediately after birth or within the first 4 hours, clinically presented by tachypnea, intercostal or subcostal retraction, wheezing, tachycardia and cyanosis.

Diagnosis based on x-ray chest as there are characteristic findings, consisting of an air bronchogram and a reticular appearance that can reach to complete opacity. Treatment is etiological by intratracheally administration of exogenous surfactant factor.

Symptomatic treatment of NRDS is based on oxygen administration and continuous positive airway pressure (CPAP) can be applied with a nasopharyngeal catheter or mechanical ventilation through a tracheal tube [70–83] (**Figures 1-3**).

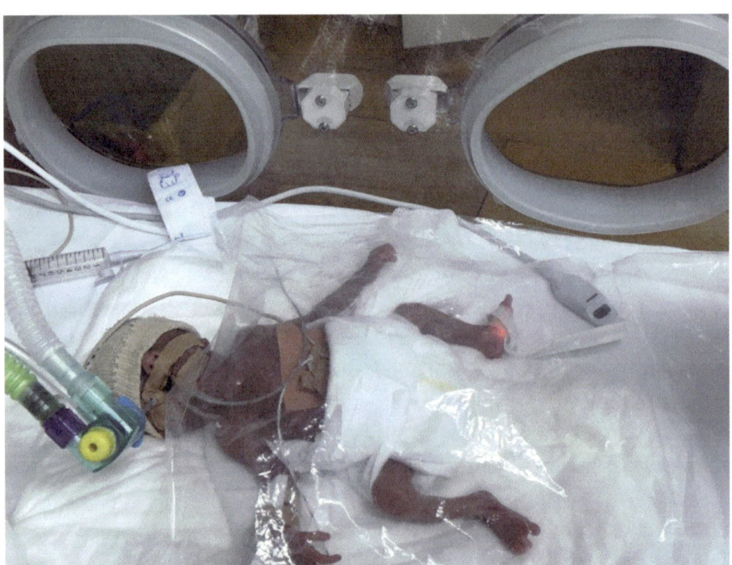

Figure 1.
Intubated neonate.

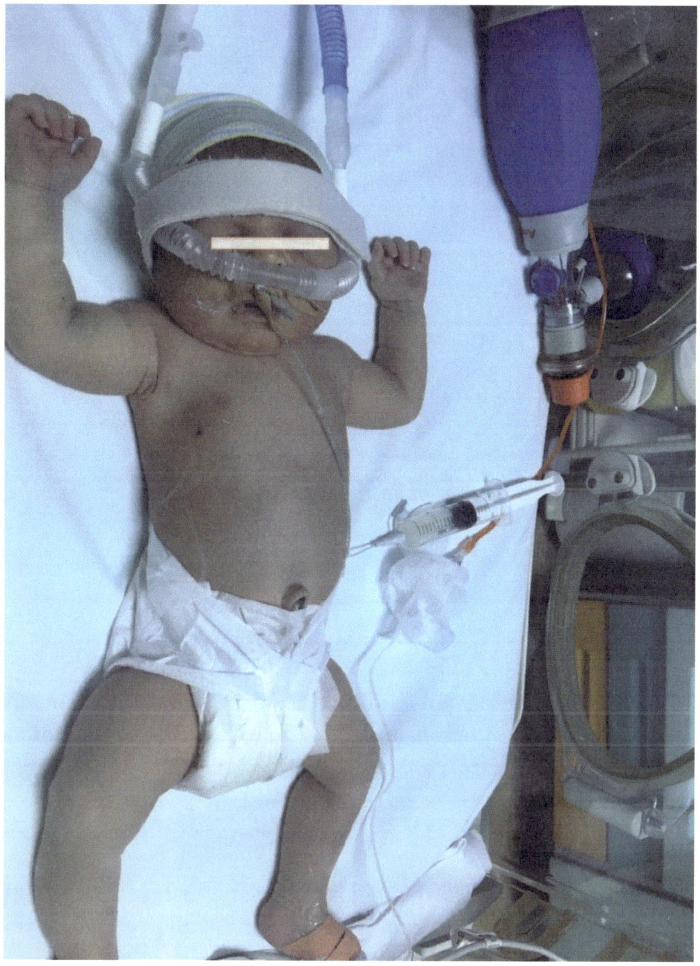

Figure 2.
CPAP in preterm neonate.

15.1.3 Apnea prematurity and bradycardia

In preterm neonates born < 32 weeks of gestation, apnea episodes are common, characterized by periods of stop breathing lasting more than 10–15 seconds, accompanied by cyanosis and bradycardia.

15.1.4 Bronchopulmonary dysplasia

Bronchopulmonary dysplasia or chronic lung disease is the most common lung disease affecting premature neonates. It is characterized by rapid and shallow breathing, dyspnea, shortness of breath, cough, and need for more oxygen. Bronchopulmonary dysplasia may be a temporary condition, but in some children, symptoms persist into adulthood, increasing the risk of developing chronic respiratory disease, such as chronic obstructive pulmonary disease (COPD) [70–83].

15.1.5 Cardiovascular disorders

These symptoms include prolonged capillary refill (>3 seconds), paleness, decreased muscle tone, lethargy, tachycardia followed by bradycardia and persistent

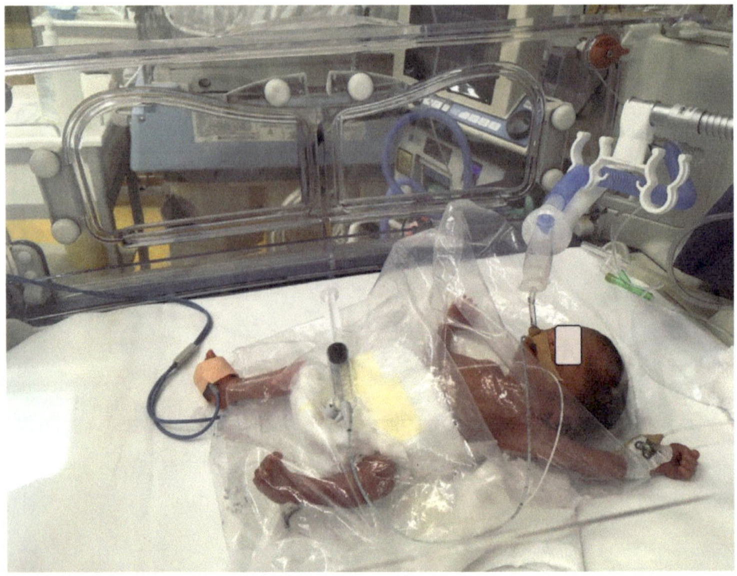

Figure 3.
Preterm neonate,weight 490 gr, 23 W.

respiratory distress, despite oxygen administration and mechanical respiratory support. In some neonates, hypotension appears from the beginning or as a late sign of shock [70–83].

15.1.6 Patent ductus arteriosus (PDA)

The major cardiovascular disorder of premature neonates is the patent ductus arteriosus stay. Its frequency reaches 25% of the total in all preterm infants and exceeds 50% in those born less than 1000 grams.

PDA may be asymptomatic or clinically presented by intense heartbeat, Corrigan pulse, and systolic or continuous murmur. If there is severe left–right escape, it causes pulmonary congestion with difficulty breathing and increased need for oxygen and mechanical respiratory support. Other manifestations include tachycardia, hepatomegaly, heart failure, and recurrent episodes of apnea. The diagnosis is based on chest X-ray which shows pulmonary edema or an increase heart shadow and on clinical examination. Finally, it is confirmed by echocardiogram, heart and large vessels Doppler. Treatment includes fluid restriction and administration of indomethacin or ibuprofen. If conservative treatment does not work then duct surgical ligation is performed [70–83].

15.1.7 Neurological disorders

Central nervous system of preterm neonates is really susceptible specifically in damages caused by labor injuries that can affect the immature intracranial structures, by the capillary bleeding, by coagulation disorders and recurrent hypoxia. It's also worth to mention the perseverance for hypoglycemia and blood pressure fluctuations that reflect in cerebral flow and pressure [70–83].

15.1.8 Neonatal brain hemorrhage

Cerebral bleed is one of the most serious problems of prematurity, as it is the commonest cause of death and disability. Its frequency is inversely proportional to gestational age and occurs in 50–60% of newborns born less than 1000 grams and in 10–20% of newborns with a birth weight of 1000 to 1500 grams [3].

The frequency has actually decreased in recent years, however, cerebral hemorrhage remain a major complication, as the survival of very preterm infants increases. 90% of brain bleeding occur in the first 3 days of life and starts in the germinal matrix, a group of immature thin-walled capillaries which is located on the head of the caudate nucleus and underneath ventricular ependyma, behind the Monroe foramen.

Size of this area is gradually decreasing, starting from 2.5 mm at 23–24 weeks to 1.4 mm at 32 weeks, and is completely regressed at 34 weeks. The diagnosis of cerebral hemorrhage and its complications based on brain ultrasound [70–83].

15.1.9 Gastrointestinal disorders

Nutrition improvement is particularly essential in the treatment of low birth weight full-term infants as well as in preterm neonates. All preterm infants are at risk due to limited nutrient stores and specific physical and developmental characteristics [70–83].

15.1.10 Necrotizing enterocolitis

The incidence of the disease in extremely preterm infants can reached 10% and the mortality in these children is about 30%. Prematurity is the most important risk factor.

The onset of the disease initiates usually within the first 10 days of life (in 90% of cases), but can range from the 1st day of life until to the 3rd month.

Symptoms in newborns vary and in mild cases recess without important sequel. Abdominal distention and lethargy are early signs of a more serious form of the disease, followed by bilious vomiting, gastrointestinal bleeding and, in severe cases, erythema of the anterior abdominal wall (especially in periumbical region).

The prognosis is actually bad and mortality rate can reach up to 20%. Bowel stenosis and malabsorption syndrome in cases of surgical resection of a large part of the intestine are some long-term complications [70–83].

15.1.11 Hematological disorders

The premature neonate is usually predisposed to hematological disorders due to increased capillary fragility, increased bleeding mood, slow red blood cell production, increased fetal hemoglobin, blood loss due to frequent peripheral blood draws and decreased albumin levels in peripheral blood. These newborns are checked for signs of bleeding at the puncture site, in the gastrointestinal tract and in the respiratory system.

15.1.12 Metabolic disorders

- Hypocalcaemia

- Hypoglycemia

  Hypoglycaemia is defined as a fall in serum glucose below 40mg/dl for preterm and full-term infants.

- Hyperglycemia

  Hyperglycemia is defined as an increase in the plasma glucose value> 130 mg/dl.

Retinopathy of prematurity
It is observed in very premature infants, who have been given oxygen in large concentrations and for a long time. After the recognition of the administered oxygen as a causative factor, the retinopathy of prematurity is now a rare disease. Newborns who are more likely to develop retinopathy are those weighing less than 1,500 grams and those who have been given oxygen in high doses for a prolonged therapy.

- Neonatal jaundice

  Jaundice is probably the most common neonatal disorder especially in premature neonates.

15.2 Preterm labor management

Maternal well-being control (infection; bleeding; WB; CRP; Urine and vaginal culture).

Fetal Well-being control (NST, US, Blood pressure, Doppler).

Corticosteroids administration if preterm labor <34 weeks is possible (betamethazone, dexamethazone) result to decrease newborn respiratory distress syndrome (50%), necrotizing enterocolitis and intraventricular hemorrhage.

Corticosteroids are contraindicated in cases of maternal sepsis.

Antibiotics: are not routinely recommended, if maternal infection is absent.

Tocolysis is recommended at least until steroids administration is completed [70–83].

15.2.1 Contraindications of tocolysis

A. Relatives

   Severe Vaginal bleeding
   Preclamspia
   Severe fetal growth restriction

B. Absolute

   Fetal death
   Fetal anomalies incompatible with life
   Chorioamnionitis
   Severe fetal distress
   Maternal indication for delivery

16. Conclusion

Despite the great progress of neonatology and prenatal medicine, prematurity is a serious factor in neonatal morbidity and mortality. Causative factors leading to prematurity have not yet been completely identified and are a really multifactorial condition. Preterm labor can be caused by a number of many different factors, such as in the case of various infections or diseases of the mother, in the absence of prenatal control, the low socio-economic level. Preterm labor is a traumatic experience and extremely stressful not only for the newborn but for the whole family.

Parents are possessed by feelings of frustration, failure as well as anxiety about the survival and future development of their baby.

The severity of a preterm birth lies in the fact that premature neonates are at greater risk for short-term and long-term complications including normal physical and mental development, disability and congenital disorders.

This is because the newborn is fully developed in the last weeks of pregnancy. That's the reason that medical and obstetric staff should contribute from the beginning of a pregnancy, in the investigation of all the causes of preterm labor in order to apply in clinical routine the appropriate treatment protocols.

Author details

Panagiotis Tsikouras[1*], Anastasia Bothou[2], Aggeliki Gerede[1], Ifigenia Apostolou[3], Fotini Gaitatzi[1], Dorelia Deuteraiou[1], Anna Chalkidou[1], Xanthoula Anthoulaki[1], Spyridon Michalopoulos[1], Georgios Dragoutsos[1], Ioannis Tsirkas[1], Irini Babageorgaka[1], Theopi Nalbanti[1], Natalia Sachnova[1], Alexios Alexiou[1], Constantinos Nikolettos[1], Apostolos Lazarou[1], Stefanos Zervoudis[1], Panagiotis Peitsidis[1] and Nikolaos Nikolettos[1]

1 Department of Obstetrics and Gynecology Democritus, University of Thrace Medical School, Alexandroupolis, Greece

2 Second Department of Surgery, Democritus University of Thrace Medical School, Alexandroupolis, Greece

3 Neonatal Intensive Unit Care, University Hospital of Thrace Medical School, Alexandroupolis, Greece

4 Technological Educational Institute of Athens and Rea Maternity Hospital, Athens, Greece

*Address all correspondence to: tsikouraspanagiotis@gmail.com

References

[1] Adams MM, Read JA, Rawlings JS, Harlass FB, Sarno AP, Rhodes PH. Preterm delivery among black and white enlisted women in the United States Army. Obstet Gynecol. 1993 Jan;81(1):65-71. PMID: 8416464

[2] Blackmore CA, Savitz DA, Edwards LJ, Harlow SD, Bowes WA Jr.Racial differences in the patterns of preterm delivery in central North Carolina, USA. Paediatr Perinat Epidemiol. 1995 Jul;9(3):281-95. doi: 10.1111/j.1365-3016.1995.tb00144.x. PMID: 7479277

[3] Schieve LA, Handler A Preterm delivery and perinatal death among black and white infants in a Chicago-area perinatal registry. Obstet Gynecol. 1996 Sep;88(3):356-63. doi: 10.1016/0029-7844(96)00203-7. PMID: 8752239

[4] Reynolds HD. Bacterial vaginosis and its implication in preterm labor and premature rupture of membranes. A review of the literature. J Nurse Midwifery. 1991 Sep-Oct;36(5):289-96. doi: 10.1016/0091-2182(91)90043-o. PMID: 1757814 Review.

[5] Newton ER. Preterm labor, preterm premature rupture of membranes, and chorioamnionitis. Clin Perinatol. 2005 Sep;32(3):571-600. doi: 10.1016/j.clp.2005.05.001. PMID: 16085021 Review.

[6] Morris JM, Roberts CL, Bowen JR, Patterson JA, Bond DM, Algert CS, Thornton JG, Crowther CA; PPROMT Collaboration. Immediate delivery compared with expectant management after preterm pre-labour rupture of the membranes close to term (PPROMT trial): a randomised controlled trial. Lancet. 2016 Jan 30;387(10017):444-52. doi: 10.1016/S0140-6736(15)00724-2. Epub 2015 Nov 10. PMID: 26564381

[7] Alexander GR, Kogan M, Bader D, Carlo W, Allen M, Mor US birth weight/gestational age-specific neonatal mortality: 1995-1997 rates for whites, hispanics, and blacks. J. Pediatrics. 2003 Jan;111(1):e61-6. doi: 10.1542/peds.111.1.e61. PMID: 12509596 Free PMC article.

[8] Alexander GR, Tompkins ME, Allen MC, Hulsey TC.Trends and racial differences in birth weight and related survival. Matern Child Health J. 1999 Jun;3(2):71-9. doi: 10.1023/a:1021849209722. PMID: 10892415

[9] Alexander GR, Kogan MD, Himes JH, Mor JM, Goldenberg R Racial differences in birthweight for gestational age and infant mortality in extremely-low-risk US populations. . Paediatr Perinat Epidemiol. 1999 Apr;13(2):205-17. doi: 10.1046/j.1365-3016.1999.00174.x. PMID: 10214610

[10] J. DeFranco EA, Hall ES, Muglia L Racial disparity in previable birth. Am J Obstet Gynecol. 2016 Mar;214(3):394.e1-7. doi: 10.1016/j.ajog.2015.12.034. Epub 2015 Dec 22. PMID: 26721776

[11] Berger TM, Bernet V, El Alama S, Fauchère JC, Hösli I, Irion O, Kind C, Latal B, Nelle M, Pfister RE, Surbek D, Truttmann AC, Wisser J, Zimmermann R. Perinatal care at the limit of viability between 22 and 26 completed weeks of gestation in Switzerland. 2011 revision of the Swiss recommendations. Swiss Med Wkly. 2011 Oct 18;141:w13280. doi: 10.4414/smw.2011.13280. eCollection 2011. PMID: 22009720 Review.

[12] Ananth CV, Friedman AM, Gyamfi-Bannerman C Epidemiology of moderate preterm, late preterm and early term delivery. Clin Perinatol. 2013 Dec;40(4):601-10. doi: 10.1016/j.clp.2013.07.001. Epub 2013 Sep 20. PMID: 24182950

[13] Chapman E, Reveiz L, Illanes E, Bonfill Cosp X. Antibiotic regimens for management of intra-amniotic infection. Cochrane Database Syst Rev. 2014 Dec 19;(12):CD010976. doi: 10.1002/14651858.CD010976.pub2. PMID: 25526426 Review.

[14] Buchanan SL, Crowther CA, Levett KM, Middleton P, Morris J. Planned early birth versus expectant management for women with preterm prelabour rupture of membranes prior to 37 weeks' gestation for improving pregnancy outcome. Cochrane Database Syst Rev. 2010 Mar 17;(3):CD004735. doi: 10.1002/14651858.CD004735.pub3. PMID: 20238332

[15] Andrews WW, Goldenberg RL; National Institute of Child Health and Human Development Maternal-Fetal Medicine Units Network. What we have learned from an antibiotic trial in fetal fibronectin positive women. Semin Perinatol. 2003 Jun;27(3):231-8. doi: 10.1016/s0146-0005(03)00006-5. PMID: 12889590 Review.

[16] Sanu O, Lamont RF. Periodontal disease and bacterial vaginosis as genetic and environmental markers for the risk of spontaneous preterm labor and preterm birth. J Matern Fetal Neonatal Med. 2011 Dec;24(12):1476-85. doi: 10.3109/14767058.2010.545930. Epub 2011 Jan 24. PMID: 21261445

[17] Beckmann M, Gardener G. Hospital versus outpatient care for preterm pre-labour rupture of membranes. Aust N Z J Obstet Gynaecol. 2013 Apr;53(2):119-24. doi: 10.1111/ajo.12021. Epub 2012 Dec 6. PMID: 23216409

[18] Faucett AM, Metz TD, DeWitt PE, Gibbs RS Effect of obesity on neonatal outcomes in pregnancies with preterm premature rupture of membranes. Am J Obstet Gynecol. 2016 Feb;214(2):287.e1-287.e5. doi: 10.1016/j.ajog.2015.09.093. Epub 2015 Oct 3. PMID: 26435047

[19] Hernández y Ballinas A, López Farán JA, Gámez Guevara C. Comparison of maternal and perinatal outcomes in the conservative treatment preterm premature membrane rupture between the use of erythromycin and clindamycin. Ginecol Obstet Mex. 2011 Jul;79(7):403-10. PMID: 21966834 Clinical Trial. Spanish.

[20] Wong LF, Holmgren CM, Silver RM, Varner MW, Manuck TA.Outcomes of expectantly managed pregnancies with multiple gestations and preterm premature rupture of membranes prior to 26 weeks. Am J Obstet Gynecol. 2015 Feb;212(2):215.e1-9. doi: 10.1016/j.ajog.2014.09.005. Epub 2014 Sep 16. PMID: 25218125 Free PMC article.

[21] Pasquier JC, Claris O, Rabilloud M, Ecochard R, Picaud JC, Moret S, Buch D, Mellier G Intentional early delivery versus expectant management for preterm premature rupture of membranes at 28-32 weeks' gestation: A multicentre randomized controlled trial (MICADO STUDY). Eur J Obstet Gynecol Reprod Biol. 2019 Feb;233:30-37. doi: 10.1016/j.ejogrb.2018.11.024. Epub 2018 Dec 5. PMID: 30553135 Clinical Trial.

[22] Gyamfi-Bannerman C. Late preterm birth: management dilemmas. Obstet Gynecol Clin North Am. 2012 Mar;39(1):35-45. doi: 10.1016/j.ogc.2011.12.005. PMID: 22370106

[23] Fuchs K, Wapner R. Elective cesarean section and induction and their impact on late preterm births. Clin Perinatol. 2006 Dec;33(4):793-801; abstract viii. doi: 10.1016/j.clp.2006.09.010. PMID: 17148005 Review.

[24] Engle WA, Kominiarek MA. Late preterm infants, early term infants, and timing of elective deliveries. Clin Perinatol. 2008 Jun;35(2):325-41, vi. doi: 10.1016/j.clp.2008.03.003. PMID: 18456072 Review.

[25] Wong AE, Grobman WA. Medically indicated--iatrogenic prematurity. Clin Perinatol. 2011 Sep;38(3):423-39. doi: 10.1016/j.clp.2011.06.002. Epub 2011 Jul 23. PMID: 21890017 Review.

[26] Meloni A, Antonelli A, Deiana S, Rocca A, Atzei A, Paoletti AM, Melis GB. Late preterm: obstetric management. J Matern Fetal Neonatal Med. 2010 Oct;23 Suppl 3:113-5. doi: 10.3109/14767058.2010.512137. PMID: 20873975

[27] Carter D. Elective early births put moms and infants at risk. Am J Nurs. 2012 Apr;112(4):19-20. doi: 10.1097/01.NAJ.0000413449.20830.f9. PMID: 22456560

[28] Goldenberg RL, Iams JD, Das A, Mercer BM, Meis PJ, Moawad AH, Miodovnik M, VanDorsten JP, Caritis SN, Thurnau GR, Dombrowski MP, Roberts JM, McNellis D. The Preterm Prediction Study: sequential cervical length and fetal fibronectin testing for the prediction of spontaneous preterm birth. National Institute of Child Health and Human Development Maternal-Fetal Medicine Units Network. Am J Obstet Gynecol. 2000 Mar;182(3):636-43. doi: 10.1067/mob.2000.104212. PMID: 10739521

[29] Goldenberg RL, Iams JD, Miodovnik M, Van Dorsten JP, Thurnau G, Bottoms S, Mercer BM, Meis PJ, Moawad AH, Das A, Caritis SN, McNellis D. The preterm prediction study: risk factors in twin gestations. National Institute of Child Health and Human Development Maternal-Fetal Medicine Units Network. Am J Obstet Gynecol. 1996 Oct;175(4 Pt 1):1047-53. doi: 10.1016/s0002-9378(96)80051-2. PMID: 8885774

[30] Goepfert AR, Goldenberg RL, Andrews WW, Hauth JC, Mercer B, Iams J, Meis P, Moawad A, Thom E, VanDorsten JP, Caritis SN, Thurnau G, Miodovnik M, Dombrowski M, Roberts J, McNellis D; National Institute of Child Health and Human Development Maternal-Fetal Medicine Units Network. The Preterm Prediction Study: association between cervical interleukin 6 concentration and spontaneous preterm birth. National Institute of Child Health and Human Development Maternal-Fetal Medicine Units Network. Am J Obstet Gynecol. 2001 Feb;184(3):483-8. doi: 10.1067/mob.2001.109653. PMID: 11228507

[31] Yu H, Wang X, Gao H, You Y, Xing A. Perinatal outcomes of pregnancies complicated by preterm premature rupture of the membranes before 34 weeks of gestation in a tertiary center in China: A retrospective review. Biosci Trends. 2015 Feb;9(1):35-41. doi: 10.5582/bst.2014.01058. PMID: 25787907 Review.

[32] Simhan HN, Canavan TP. Preterm premature rupture of membranes: diagnosis, evaluation and management strategies. BJOG. 2005 Mar;112 Suppl 1:32-7. doi: 10.1111/j.1471-0528.2005.00582.x. PMID: 15715592 Review.

[33] Tsikouras P, Anastasopoulos G, Maroulis V, Bothou A, Chalkidou A, Deuteraiou D, Anthoulaki X, Tsatsaris G, Bourazan AH, Iatrakis G, Zervoudis S, Galazios G, Inagamova LK, Csorba R, Teichmann AT. Comparative Evaluation of Arabin Pessary and Cervical Cerclage for the Prevention of Preterm Labor in Asymptomatic Women with High Risk Factors. Int J Environ Res Public Health. 2018 Apr 18;15(4):791. doi: 10.3390/ijerph15040791. PMID: 29670041

[34] Sieroszewski P, Jasiński A, Perenc M, Banach R, Oszukowski P. The Arabin pessary for the treatment of threatened mid-trimester miscarriage or premature labour and miscarriage: a case series. J Matern Fetal Neonatal Med. 2009 Jun;22(6):469-72. doi:

10.1080/14767050802531748. PMID: 19530009 Clinical Trial.

[35] Barinov SV, Shamina IV, Lazareva OV, Tirskaya YI, Ralko VV, Shkabarnya LL, Dikke GB, Kochev DM, Klementyeva LL. Comparative assessment of arabin pessary, cervical cerclage and medical management for preterm birth prevention in high-risk pregnancies. J Matern Fetal Neonatal Med. 2017 Aug;30(15):1841-1846. doi: 10.1080/14767058.2016.1228054. Epub 2016 Sep 9. PMID: 27550418

[36] Ting YH, Lao TT, Wa Law L, Hui SY, Chor CM, Lau TK, Yeung Leung T. Arabin cerclage pessary in the management of cervical insufficiency. J Matern Fetal Neonatal Med. 2012 Dec;25(12):2693-5. doi: 10.3109/14767058.2012.712559. Epub 2012 Aug 22. PMID: 22871155

[37] Boelig RC, Berghella V. Current options for mechanical prevention of preterm birth. Semin Perinatol. 2017 Dec;41(8):452-460. doi: 10.1053/j.semperi.2017.08.003. Epub 2017 Oct 13. PMID: 29033106 Review.

[38] Saccone G, Ciardulli A, Xodo S, Dugoff L, Ludmir J, Pagani G, Visentin S, Gizzo S, Volpe N, Maruotti GM, Rizzo G, Martinelli P, Berghella V.Cervical Pessary for Preventing Preterm Birth in Singleton Pregnancies With Short Cervical Length: A Systematic Review and Meta-analysis. J Ultrasound Med. 2017 Aug;36(8):1535-1543. doi: 10.7863/ultra.16.08054. Epub 2017 Apr 11. PMID: 28398701

[39] Bonanno C, Wapner RJ. Antenatal corticosteroids in the management of preterm birth: are we back where we started? Obstet Gynecol Clin North Am. 2012 Mar;39(1):47-63. doi: 10.1016/j.ogc.2011.12.006. PMID: 22370107

[40] Briceño-Pérez C, Reyna-Villasmil E, Vigil-De-Gracia P. Antenatal corticosteroid therapy: Historical and scientific basis to improve preterm birth management. . Eur J Obstet Gynecol Reprod Biol. 2019 Mar;234:32-37. doi: 10.1016/j.ejogrb.2018.12.025. Epub 2019 Jan 6. PMID: 30639954 Review.

[41] Fuchs F, Audibert F, Senat MV. Prenatal corticosteroids: short-term and long-term effects of multiple courses. Literature review in 2013. J Gynecol Obstet Biol Reprod (Paris). 2014 Mar;43(3):211-7. doi: 10.1016/j.jgyn.2013.11.015. Epub 2014 Feb 12. PMID: 24529761 Review. French.

[42] Crowther CA, Ashwood P, Andersen CC, Middleton PF, Tran T, Doyle LW, Robinson JS, Harding JE; ASTEROID Study Group.Maternal intramuscular dexamethasone versus betamethasone before preterm birth (ASTEROID): a multicentre, double-blind, randomised controlled trial. Lancet Child Adolesc Health. 2019 Nov;3(11):769-780. doi: 10.1016/S2352-4642(19)30292-5. Epub 2019 Sep 12. PMID: 31523039 Clinical Trial.

[43] Hong S, Lee SM, Kwak DW, Lee J, Kim SY, Oh JW, Oh S, Park CW, Park JS, Chung JH, Jun JK. Effects of antenatal corticosteroids in twin neonates with late preterm birth (ACTWIN [Antenatal Corticosteroids in TWIN late preterm neonates] trial): study protocol for a randomized controlled trial. BMC Pregnancy Childbirth. 2019 Apr 3;19(1):114. doi: 10.1186/s12884-019-2235-5. PMID: 30943910 Free PMC article.

[44] Hong S, Lee SM, Kwak DW, Lee J, Kim SY, Oh JW, Oh S, Park CW, Park JS, Chung JH, Jun JK. Schmitz T. Prevention of preterm birth complications by antenatal corticosteroid administration. J Gynecol Obstet Biol Reprod (Paris). 2016 Dec;45(10):1399-1417. doi: 10.1016/j.jgyn.2016.09.008. Epub 2016 Oct 21. PMID: 27776846 Review

[45] Mercer B. Antibiotics in the management of PROM and preterm labor. . Obstet Gynecol Clin North Am. 2012 Mar;39(1):65-76. doi: 10.1016/j.ogc.2011.12.007. Epub 2012 Jan 28. PMID: 22370108

[46] Jackson GL, Rawiki P, Sendelbach D, Manning MD, Engle WD. Hospital course and short-term outcomes of term and late preterm neonates following exposure to prolonged rupture of membranes and/or chorioamnionitis. Pediatr Infect Dis J. 2012 Jan;31(1):89-90. doi: 10.1097/INF.0b013e31822fb15d. PMID: 21860336

[47] Hernández y Ballinas A, López Farán JA, Gámez Guevara C. Comparison of maternal and perinatal outcomes in the conservative treatment preterm premature membrane rupture between the use of erythromycin and clindamycin. Ginecol Obstet Mex. 2011 Jul;79(7):403-10. PMID: 21966834 Clinical Trial. Spanish.

[48] Ovalle A, Romero R, Gómez R, Martínez MA, Nien JK, Ferrand P, Aspillaga C, Figueroa J. Antibiotic administration to patients with preterm labor and intact membranes: is there a beneficial effect in patients with endocervical inflammation? . J Matern Fetal Neonatal Med. 2006 Aug;19(8):453-64. doi: 10.1080/14767050600852668. PMID: 16966109 Clinical Trial.

[49] Newton ER. Preterm labor, preterm premature rupture of membranes, and chorioamnionitis. Clin Perinatol. 2005 Sep;32(3):571-600. doi: 10.1016/j.clp.2005.05.001. PMID: 16085021 Review.

[50] Singh K, Mercer B. Antibiotics after preterm premature rupture of the membranes. Clin Obstet Gynecol. 2011 Jun;54(2):344-50. doi: 10.1097/GRF.0b013e318217ec5d. PMID: 21508705

[51] Mothers' experiences of parenting and everyday life of children born at 23 weeks of gestation - a qualitative descriptive study. Väliaho A, Lehtonen L, Axelin A, Korja R. BMC Pediatr. 2021 Jan 23;21(1):48. doi: 10.1186/s12887-020-02478-y. PMID: 33485315 Free PMC article.

[52] An Initiative to Reduce Preterm Infants Pre-discharge Growth Failure Through Time-specific Feeding Volume Increase. Chu SS, White HO, Rindone SL, Tripp SA, Rhein LM. Pediatr Qual Saf. 2020 Dec 28;6(1):e366. doi: 10.1097/pq9.0000000000000366. eCollection 2021 Jan-Feb. PMID: 33403313

[53] Ozkur M, Dogulu F, Ozkur A, Gokmen B, Inaloz SS, Aynacioglu AS. Association of the Gln27Glu polymorphism of the beta-2-adrenergic receptor with preterm labor. Int J Gynaecol Obstet. 2002 Jun;77(3):209-15. doi: 10.1016/s0020-7292(02)00035-8. PMID: 12065131

[54] Landau R. Genetic contributions to labor pain and progress. Clin Perinatol. 2013 Sep;40(3):575-87. doi: 10.1016/j.clp.2013.05.014. Epub 2013 Jun 27. PMID: 23972758 Review.

[55] Landau R, Liu SK, Blouin JL, Carvalho B. The effect of OPRM1 and COMT genotypes on the analgesic response to intravenous fentanyl labor analgesia. Anesth Analg. 2013 Feb;116(2):386-91. doi: 10.1213/ANE.0b013e318273f2c7. Epub 2013 Jan 9. PMID: 23302985

[56] Song Z, Du B, Wang K, Shi X. Effects of OPRM1 A118G polymorphism on epidural analgesia with fentanyl during labor: a meta-analysis. Genet Test Mol Biomarkers. 2013 Oct;17(10):743-9. doi: 10.1089/gtmb.2013.0282. Epub 2013 Aug 2. PMID: 23909491 Review.

[57] Hannah C Glass, Andrew T Costarino, Stephen A Stayer, Claire M

Brett, Franklyn Cladis, Peter J Davis Outcomes for extremely premature infants PMID: 25988638 PMCID: PMC4438860

[58] Salverda HH, Oldenburger NJ, Rijken M, Pauws SC, Dargaville PA, Te Pas AB. The effect of automated oxygen control on clinical outcomes in preterm infants: a pre- and post-implementation cohort study. Eur J Pediatr. 2021 Feb 23. doi: 10.1007/s00431-021-03982-8. Online ahead of print. PMID: 33619593

[59] Early protein intake predicts functional connectivity and neurocognition in preterm born children. Duerden EG, Thompson B, Poppe T, Alsweiler J, Gamble G, Jiang Y, Leung M, Tottman AC, Wouldes T, Miller SP, Harding JE; PIANO study group. Sci Rep. 2021 Feb 18;11(1):4085. doi: 10.1038/s41598-021-83125-z. PMID: 33602973 Free PMC article.

[60] Precordial ECG Amplitudes in the Days After Birth: Electrocardiographic Changes During Transition from Fetal to Neonatal Circulation. Hvidemose SO, Pærregaard MM, Pihl CA, Pietersen AH, Iversen KK, Bundgaard H, Christensen AH. Pediatr Cardiol. 2021 Jan 28. doi: 10.1007/s00246-021-02547-8. Online ahead of print. PMID: 33507333

[61] Salafia CM, Minior VK, Pezzullo JC, Popek EJ, Rosenkrantz TS, Vintzileos AM. Intrauterine growth restriction in infants of less than thirty-two weeks' gestation: associated placental pathologic features. Am J Obstet Gynecol. 1995 Oct;173(4):1049-57. doi: 10.1016/0002-9378(95)91325-4. PMID: 7485292

[62] Gargano JW, Holzman CB, Senagore PK, Reuss ML, Pathak DR, Friderici KH, Jernigan K, Fisher R. Polymorphisms in thrombophilia and renin-angiotensin system pathways, preterm delivery, and evidence of placental hemorrhage. Am J Obstet Gynecol. 2009 Sep;201(3):317.e1-9. doi: 10.1016/j.ajog.2009.05.060. PMID: 19733287

[63] Nemeth E, Millar LK, Bryant-Greenwood G. Fetal membrane distention: II. Differentially expressed genes regulated by acute distention in vitro. Am J Obstet Gynecol. 2000 Jan;182(1 Pt 1):60-7. doi: 10.1016/s0002-9378(00)70491-1. PMID: 10649157

[64] Genetics of the cervix in relation to preterm birth. Warren JE, Silver RM. Semin Perinatol. 2009 Oct;33(5):308-11. doi: 10.1053/j.semperi.2009.06.003. PMID: 19796727 Review

[65] Shanbhag S, Clark H, Timmaraju V, Bhattacharya S, Cruickshank M. Pregnancy outcome after treatment for cervical intraepithelial neoplasia. Obstet Gynecol. 2009 Oct;114(4):727-735. doi: 10.1097/AOG.0b013e3181b5cba3. PMID: 19888028

[66] Pettersson FD, Grönbladh A, Nyberg F, Sundström-Poromaa I, Åkerud H. The A118G single-nucleotide polymorphism of human μ-opioid receptor gene and use of labor analgesia. Reprod Sci. 2012 Sep;19(9):962-7. doi: 10.1177/1933719112438970. Epub 2012 Apr 23. PMID: 22527985

[67] Sweet DG, Carnielli V, Greisen G, Hallman M, Ozek E, Plavka R, Saugstad OD, Simeoni U, Speer CP, Vento M, Halliday HL; European consensus guidelines on the management of neonatal respiratory distress syndrome in preterm infants--2013 update. European Association of Perinatal Medicine. Neonatology. 2013;103(4):353-68. doi: 10.1159/000349928. Epub 2013 May 31. PMID: 23736015

[68] Sweet DG, Carnielli V, Greisen G, Hallman M, Ozek E, Plavka R, Saugstad OD, Simeoni U, Speer CP, Halliday HL; European consensus

guidelines on the management of neonatal respiratory distress syndrome in preterm infants - 2010 update. European Association of Perinatal Medicine. Neonatology. 2010 Jun;97(4):402-17. doi: 10.1159/000297773. Epub 2010 Jun 10. PMID: 20551710

[69] Sweet D, Bevilacqua G, Carnielli V, Greisen G, Plavka R, Saugstad OD, Simeoni U, Speer CP, Valls-I-Soler A, Halliday H; European consensus guidelines on the management of neonatal respiratory distress syndrome. Working Group on Prematurity of the World Association of Perinatal Medicine; European Association of Perinatal Medicine. J Perinat Med. 2007;35(3):175-86. doi: 10.1515/JPM.2007.048. PMID: 17480144

[70] Sweet DG, Carnielli V, Greisen G, Hallman M, Ozek E, Te Pas A, Plavka R, Roehr CC, Saugstad OD, Simeoni U, Speer CP, Vento M, Visser GHA, Halliday HL European Consensus Guidelines on the Management of Respiratory Distress Syndrome - 2019 Update. . Neonatology. 2019;115(4):432-450. doi: 10.1159/000499361. Epub 2019 Apr 11. PMID: 30974433 Free PMC article.

[71] Sweet DG, Carnielli V, Greisen G, Hallman M, Ozek E, Plavka R, Saugstad OD, Simeoni U, Speer CP, Vento M, Visser GH, Halliday HL. European Consensus Guidelines on the Management of Respiratory Distress Syndrome - 2016 Update. Neonatology. 2017;111(2):107-125. doi: 10.1159/000448985. Epub 2016 Sep 21. PMID: 27649091

[72] Rodriguez RJ. Management of respiratory distress syndrome: an update. Respir Care. 2003 Mar;48(3):279-86; discussion 286-7. PMID: 12667277 Review.

[73] Low JA, Wood SL, Killen HL, Pater EA, Karchmar EJ. Intrapartum asphyxia in the preterm fetus less than 2000 gm. Am J Obstet Gynecol. 1990 Feb;162(2):378-82. doi: 10.1016/0002-9378(90)90390-s. PMID: 2309819

[74] Low JA, Pickersgill H, Killen H, Derrick EJ. The prediction and prevention of intrapartum fetal asphyxia in term pregnancies. Am J Obstet Gynecol. 2001 Mar;184(4):724-30. doi: 10.1067/mob.2001.111720. PMID: 11262479

[75] Low JA, Pancham SR, Piercy WN, Worthington D, Karchmar J. Intrapartum fetal asphyxia: clinical characteristics, diagnosis, and significance in relation to pattern of development. Am J Obstet Gynecol. 1977 Dec 15;129(8):857-72. doi: 10.1016/0002-9378(77)90519-1. PMID: 22248

[76] Low JA, Panagiotopoulos C, Derrick EJ. Newborn complications after intrapartum asphyxia with metabolic acidosis in the preterm fetus. Am J Obstet Gynecol. 1995 Mar;172(3):805-10. doi: 10.1016/0002-9378(95)90003-9. PMID: 7892868

[77] Low JA. Intrapartum fetal asphyxia: definition, diagnosis, and classification. Am J Obstet Gynecol. 1997 May;176(5):957-9. doi: 10.1016/s0002-9378(97)70385-5. PMID: 9166151 Review.

[78] Low JA. The relationship of asphyxia in the mature fetus to long-term neurologic function. Clin Obstet Gynecol. 1993 Mar;36(1):82-90. doi: 10.1097/00003081-199303000-00011. PMID: 8435949 Review.Anesth Analg 1994 May;78(5):912-7. doi: 10.1213/00000539-199405000-00013.

[79] S H Rolbin, M M Cohen, C M Levinton, E N Kelly, D Farine. The premature infant: anesthesia for cesarean delivery PMID: 8160989 DOI: 10.1213/00000539-199405000-00013

[80] Nwafor MI, Aniebue UU, Nwankwo TO, Onyeka TC, Okafor VU. Perinatal outcome of preterm cesarean section in a resource-limited centre: a comparison between general anaesthesia and subarachnoid block. Niger J Clin Pract. 2014 Sep-Oct;17(5):613-8. doi: 10.4103/1119-3077.141428. PMID: 25244273

[81] Levy BT, Dawson JD, Toth PP, Bowdler N. Predictors of neonatal resuscitation, low Apgar scores, and umbilical artery pH among growth-restricted neonates. Obstet Gynecol. 1998 Jun;91(6):909-16. doi: 10.1016/s0029-7844(98)00094-5. PMID: 9610995

[82] Ong BY, Cohen MM, Palahniuk RJ. Anesthesia for cesarean section--effects on neonates. Anesth Analg. 1989 Mar;68(3):270-5. PMID: 2919765

[83] Burguet A, Pez O, Debaene B, Untersteller M, Bettinger G, Kayemba-Kays S, Thiriez G, Bouthet MF, Sanyas P, Menget A, Mulin B, Maillet R, Boisselier P, Pierre F, Gouyon JB. Very preterm birth: is maternal anesthesia a risk factor for neonatal intubation in the delivery room?. Arch Pediatr. 2009 Dec;16(12):1547-53. doi: 10.1016/j.arcped.2009.09.011. Epub 2009 Oct 23. PMID: 19854034 French.

Section 3

Papillary Neoplasm and Melanoma

Chapter 5

Papillary Neoplasm of Breast-Changing Trends in Diagnosis and Management

Amrit Pal Singh Rana and Manjit Kaur Rana

Abstract

Papillary neoplasm of breast comprises of seven separate heterogeneous entities ranging from benign, atypical and malignancy including non-invasive and invasive carcinoma. Papillary carcinoma (PC) is seen more commonly in older postmenopausal women with favorable prognosis. PC breast typically presents with bloody nipple discharge and an abnormal mass with radiologic features of intraductal mass. Encapsulated PC and solid PC is to be treated as in situ carcinoma, but distinction of invasive PC from non invasive carcinoma is critical both at microscopic and molecular level. So, surgical excision should be the choice of definitive diagnostic technique in papillary neoplasm instead of core needle biopsy. Furthermore, treatment guidelines for invasive PC also have been framed, but incidence of recurrence and death attributable to various subtypes of carcinoma remained same. So, this is important topic to be addressed to understand the need for further management and outcome of the disease.

Keywords: papilloma, invasive carcinoma, intraductal, carcinoma in situ, solid papillary carcinoma

1. Introduction

Papillary neoplasm of the breast is a broad range of heterogeneous group of lesions that are characterized by presence of papillae supported by fibrovascular cores lined by epithelial cells with or without myoepithelial cell layer. These neoplasms may be benign, atypical or malignant and are difficult to diagnose. The main diagnostic concern is differentiating benign and malignant lesions, which can be challenging both on imaging as well as on histopathological examination [1].

2. Definition of papillary neoplasm breast

World health organization (WHO) in 2021 classified breast intraductal papillary neoplasm as intraductal papillomas (intraductal papilloma with atypical hyperplasia, intraductal papilloma with ductual carcinoma in situ (DCIS), intraductal papilloma with lobular carcinoma in situ), intraductal papillary carcinoma (solid papillary carcinoma, encapsulated carcinoma) and invasive carcinoma [1, 2].

3. Epidemiology

3.1 Age and sex

The benign conditions are commonly seen in between 30 and 50 years of age and PC commonly affects postmenopausal age group. Papillary neoplasms have sex predilection for females though intracystic papillary carcinoma (IPC) is rarely seen in males too. The clinical presentation in males and females is similar except for a higher median age in males [3, 4].

3.2 Incidence

Papillary neoplasms are less commonly seen and account for less than 3% of breast tumors and PC of the breast accounts for 0.5–1% of breast cancer [5]. The frequency of lymph node involvement in invasive papillary carcinoma, its local recurrence and distant recurrence may be 0–11%, 3–70% and 0–4%, respectively. Solid papillary carcinoma (SPC) constitutes only 1% of all the breast carcinomas, presenting as localized mass in approximately 90% of the cases, lymph node metastases in 8%, and distant metastases in less than 0.8% only. Intracystic papillary carcinoma also has localized involvement in approximately 89.6% of the cases with 0.4% distant metastases [6, 7].

4. Pathophysiology

Many researchers have analyzed the risk factors for malignant transformation in benign papilloma of breast, however the results remain inconsistent. Some investigators considered same attributable factors for carcinoma arising in papillary neoplasm as that of other carcinomas. The contributing predisposing risk factors are age, family history, genetic predilection, diet and weight gain, alcoholism, and endocrine factors [8, 9].

5. Clinical features

Papillary neoplasms may be central and peripheral in location and solitary or multiple in number. And most papillomas are centrally located with a wide age distribution and originate in the large ducts, and are typically solitary. The most common clinical presentation is serous or serosanguineous nipple discharge. The benign solitary papilloma has 1.5 to 2.0 times high risk of breast carcinoma whereas four times increased risk of malignant transformation is noted in atypical papillomas. The peripheral papillomas arise in the terminal duct lobular units and are often discovered incidentally on imaging studies and risk of carcinoma is even higher than solitary papilloma. And very rarely, benign papillomas of breast presenting with local or distant metastases have been reported [10–18]. However, behavior and management of papillary carcinoma whether in situ or invasive remain a matter of debate. The lymph node involvement, local recurrence and distant recurrence may be seen. Solid papillary carcinoma are localized lesions and may involve lymph node however distant metastasis is rare [6, 7]. Common clinical features include nipple discharge and palpable masses in some cases, however papillary lesions may be diagnosed in asymptomatic women or on screening [19].

6. Diagnosis

Treatment of benign papillary neoplasms require careful evaluation as the presence of papillary architecture is known to be associated with a higher risk of carcinoma breast [20]. The precise diagnosis of papillary neoplasm of the breast is difficult on cytomorphological charaterstics alone. A benign diagnosis on fine needle aspiration or core needle biopsy may not completely exclude malignancy especially if it manifests as focal carcinoma in-situ or abruption of the myoepithelial layer. Microcalcification is an important factor in the management of breast intraductal papillomas diagnosed on core biopsy [21–24]. The benign papillary lesions can be diagnosed with sonographically guided 14-gauge core needle biopsy. The sensitivity for detecting papillary lesions is greater by ultrasound than mammography. The USG findings of papillary neoplasm are found to be correlated with pathologic findings [13, 25]. Recently, automated breast ultrasound scanners have been developed, and the ultrasound volume data set of the whole breast can be acquired in a standard manner [26]. MRI features including a mass size exceeding 10 mm may indicate a papilloma with high-risk or malignant lesions [27].

However, histopathological examination is the gold standard tool for the diagnosis. Nevertheless, the morphology is more important than the immunostaining pattern, and diagnosis of neoplastic proliferation should not be made on the immunostaining pattern alone. For intraductal papillary neoplasm CK5/6 is good marker to differentiate between intraductal hyperplasia (CK5/6 positive) and intraductal proliferation resembling DCIS or ADH (CK5/6 negative). Immunohistochemical examination with CK5/6 and a panel of two myoepithelial markers (p63, SMA, CD10, calponin) acts as useful tool in assessing papillary neoplasms of the breast [28, 29].

7. Treatment and prognosis

The treatment of benign and atypical papilloma is being evolved. The surgical excision of all papillary lesions is recommended for definitive diagnosis and standard management for malignant papillary lesions [24, 30]. Li X et al. suggested the vacuum assisted excision is applicable for complete excision of small papillomas, even papillomas with atypical hyperplasia [31]. Bianchi et al. also emphasized that, in addition to surgery, vacuum assisted excision of beingn intraductal papilloma may be done [32]. However, some authors have recommended that benign papillary lesions diagnosed by core needle biopsy (CNB) might not require immediate excision, but may be safely managed with imaging follow-up for at least 5 years rather than with surgical excision [33, 34]. Accurate results and coordination between a trained radiologist and pathology are of utmost importance in the decision making between follow-up or surgery [35]. However, Fatima K et al. have observed no reliable clinical or imaging features that can pre-surgically predict atypical upgradation or malignant potential [30]. Tokiniwa H and fellows detected surgical excision advantageous for papillary lesions especially for the lesions located far from the nipple [36]. The atypical papillary lesions should be excised surgically (**Figure 1**) [37].

Intraductal carcinomas like encapsulated papillary carcinoma (EPC) with presence of myoepithelial cells at the periphery should be treated as DCIS and with lack of myoepithelial cells may behave in an indolent invasive pattern with reported lymphnode metastasis and lymphovascular invasion. The present harmony is to manage EPC as in situ disease, though recurrence may be seen associated with aggressive behavior (**Figure 2**).

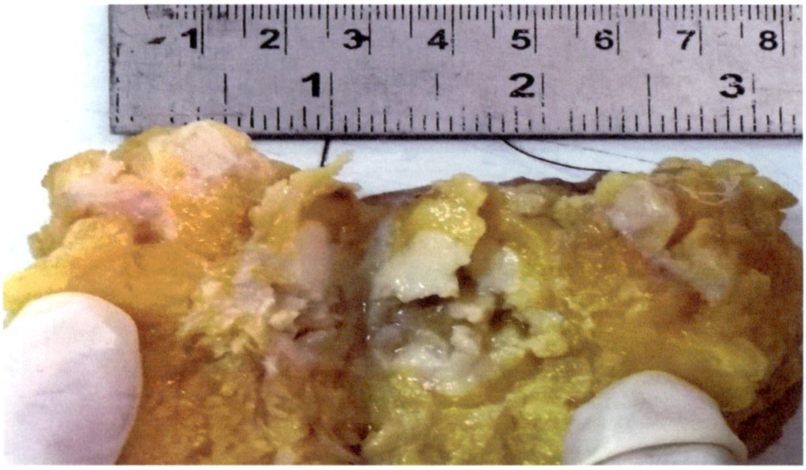

Figure 1.
Surgically excised specimen of papillary neoplasm.

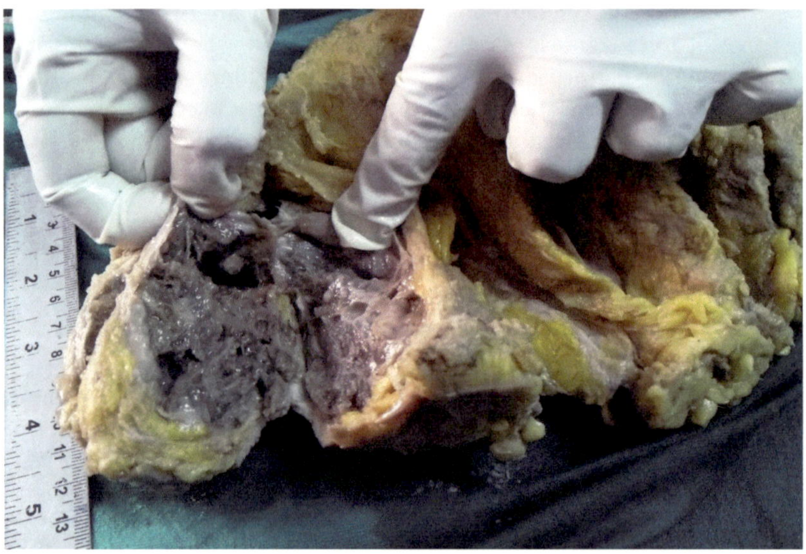

Figure 2.
Surgically excised specimen of EPC.

Due to lack of evidence of behavior and criterion of diagnosis, SPC is difficult to categorize as benign or malignant and current consensus is to consider it as an in-situ disease. Consensus is to treat these types of neoplasms for local control without axillary node sampling or systemic therapy. Inspite of very low risk of metastatic potential, evidence does not support use of conventional forms of adjuvant systemic therapy. IPC is known to have benign behavior with 100% disease-specific survival rate so to be treated with similar way to other types of carcinoma breast except in cases with moderate nuclear atypia [7, 38].

8. Conclusion

Papillary neoplasm is difficult to detect and diagnose, if diagnosed, surgical excision is the treatment of choice. Encysted and solid papillary carcinoma should be treated as DCIS, irrespective of nuclear grading. Amongst imaging studies ultrasoography is better than mammography. In difficult cases immunohistochemical markers (CK 5/6 and minimum two myeloepithelial markers provide the support. Invasive papillary carcinoma may be treated as per guidelines of invasive carcinoma breast and shows good prognosis.

Author details

Amrit Pal Singh Rana[1*] and Manjit Kaur Rana[2]

1 Department of Surgery, Baba Farid University of Health Sciences, Faridkot, Punjab, India

2 Department of Pathology/Lab Medicine, All India Institute of Medical Sciences, Bathinda, Punjab, India

*Address all correspondence to: dramritpalsingh@gmail.com

References

[1] Tan PH, Schnitt SJ, van de Vijver MJ, Ellis IO, Lakhani SR. Papillary and neuroendocrine breast lesions: The WHO stance. Histopathology. 2015;66(6):761-770.

[2] Basavaiah SH, Minal J, Sreeram S, et al. Diagnostic pitfalls in papillary lesions of the breast: Experience from a single tertiary care center. J Clin. Diagn. Res. 2016;10(8):EC18–EC21.

[3] Arora R, Gupta R, Sharma A, Dinda AK. Invasive papillary carcinoma of male breast. Indian J Pathol Microbiol. 2010 Jan-Mar; 53(1):135-137.

[4] Zhao Y, Li N, Gong X, Yu L, Jin X. Clinicopathologic features of intraductal papillary neoplasm of breast: Analyses of three cases. Int J Clin Exp Pathol. 2017;10(9):9575-9582.

[5] Kuehner G, Darbinian J, Habel L, et al. Benign papillary breast mass lesions: Favorable outcomes with surgical excision or imaging surveillance. Ann. Surg. Oncol. 2019;26(6):1695-1703.

[6] Guo S, Wang Y, Rohr J, Fan C, Li Q, Li X, Wang Z. Solid papillary carcinoma of the breast: A special entity needs to be distinguished from conventional invasive carcinoma avoiding over-treatment. Breast. 2016;26:67-72.

[7] Rakha EA, Gandhi N, Climent F, van Deurzen CH, Haider SA, Dunk L, Lee AH, Macmillan D, Ellis IO. Encapsulated papillary carcinoma of the breast: An invasive tumor with excellent prognosis. Am J Surg Pathol. 2011 Aug; 35(8):1093-1103.

[8] Shiino S, Tsuda H, Yoshida M, Jimbo K, Asaga S, Hojo T and Kinoshita T. Intraductal papillomas on core biopsy can be upgraded to malignancy on subsequent excisional biopsy regardless of the presence of atypical features. Pathol Int. 2015; 65:293-300.

[9] Zhu Y, Zhang S, Liu P, Lu H, Xu Y and Yang WT. Solitary intraductal papillomas of the breast: MRI features and differentiation from small invasive ductal carcinomas. AJR Am J Roentgenol. 2012;199:936-942.

[10] Han S-H, Kim M, Chung YR, et al. Benign intraductal papilloma without atypia on core needle biopsy has a low rate of upgrading to malignancy after excision. J Breast Cancer 2018;21:80-86.

[11] Greif F, Sharon E, Shechtman I, Morgenstern S, Gutman H. Eur. Carcinoma within solitary ductal papilloma of the breast. J Surg Oncol. 2010 Apr; 36(4):384-6.)

[12] Muttarak M, Lerttumnongtum P, Chaiwun B, et al. Spectrum of papillary lesions of the breast: Clinical, imaging, and pathologic correlation. Am J Roentgenol 2008;191:700-707.

[13] Eiada R, Chong J, Kulkarni S, et al. Papillary lesions of the breast: MRI, ultrasound, and mammographic appearances. Am J Roentgenol. 2012;198:264-271.

[14] Khan S, Diaz A, Archer KJ, Lehman RR, Mullins T, Cardenosa G, Bear HD. Papillary lesions of the breast: To excise or observe? Breast J. 2018;24(3):350-355.

[15] Singh T, Tso E, Kumar A, Ahrens P. Axillary lymph node metastases from papilloma of the breast [abstract]. J Clin Oncol. 2006;24(18):10764.

[16] Dzodic R, Stanojevic B, Saenko V, Nakashima M, Markovic I, Pupic G, et al. Intraductal papilloma of ectopic breast tissue in axillary lymph node of a patient with a previous intraductal

papilloma of ipsilateral breast: A case report and review of the literature. Diagn Pathol. 2010;5:17. DOI:10.1186/1746-1596-5-17.

[17] Cottom H, Rengabashyam B, Turton PE, Shaaban AM. Intraductal papilloma in an axillary lymph node of a patient with human immunodeficiency virus: A case report and review of the literature. J Med Case Rep. 2014;8:162. DOI:10.1186/1752-1947-8-162.

[18] Jain AL, Mullins J, Smith JR, et al. Unusual recurrent metastasizing benign breast papilloma: A case report. J Med Case Rep. 2020;14(1):33. Published 2020 Feb 19. DOI:10.1186/s13256-020-2354-7)

[19] Hong YR, Song BJ, Jung SS, Kang BJ, Kim SH, Chae BJ. Predictive factors for upgrading patients with benign breast papillary lesions using a core needle biopsy. J. Breast Cancer. 2016;19(4): 410-416.

[20] Choi SH, Jo S, Kim D-H, et al. Clinical and imaging characteristics of papillary neoplasms of the breast associated with malignancy: A retrospective cohort study. Ultrasound Med Biol. 2014; 40:2599-2608.

[21] Prathiba D, Rao S, Kshitija K, Joseph LD. Papillary lesions of breast – An introspect of cytomorphological features. J Cytol. 2010;27(1):12-15. DOI:10.4103/0970-9371.66692

[22] Collins L, Schnitt S. Papillary lesions of the breast: Selected diagnostic and management issues. Histopathology 2008;52:20-29.

[23] Lam WWM, Chu WCW, Tang APY, et al. Role of radiologic features in the management of papillary lesions of the breast. Am J Roentgenol 2006;186: 1322-1327.

[24] Hassan T, Delli Fraine P, El-Khoury M, Joseph L, Zheng J, Mesurolle B. Surgical follow-up and clinical presentation of 142 breast papillary lesions diagnosed by ultrasound-guided core-needle biopsy. J Clin Ultrasound. 2013;41(1):1-9.

[25] Brookes MJ, Bourke AG. Radiological appearances of papillary breast lesions. Clin Radiol. 2008 Nov; 63(11):1265-1273.

[26] Kelly KM, Dean J, Comulada WS, Lee SJ. Breast cancer detection using automated whole breast ultrasound and mammography in radiographically dense breasts. Eur Radiol. 2010;20:734-742. DOI:10.1007/s00330-009-1588-y

[27] Wang LJ, Wu P, Li XX, Luo R, Wang DB, Guan WB. Magnetic resonance imaging features for differentiating breast papilloma with high-risk or malignant lesions from benign papilloma: A retrospective study on 158 patients. World J Surg Oncol. 2018;16(1):234. DOI:10.1186/s12957-018-1537-9)10.1186/s12957-018-1537-9)

[28] Tse GM, Tan PH, Moriya T. The role of immunohistochemistry in the differential diagnosis of papillary lesions of the breast. J Clin Pathol. 2009; 62(5):407-413.

[29] Omi Y, Yamamoto T, Okamoto T, Obara T, Kobayashi M. A useful immunohistochemical approach to evaluate intraductal proliferative lesions of the breast and to predict their prognosis. Histol Histopathol. 2011;26(1):79-86.

[30] Fatima K, Afzal S, Tariq MU. Outcome of non-malignant papillary lesions of the breast on core biopsy: An experience from a tertiary care center in Pakistan. Cureus. 2020;12(5):e8364.

[31] Li X, Gao H, Xu M, Wu Y, Gao D. Breast papillary lesions diagnosed and treated using ultrasound-guided vacuum-assisted excision. BMC Surg. 2020;20(1):204. DOI:10.1186/s12893-020-00869-7

[32] Bianchi S, Bendinelli B, Saladino V, et al. Non-malignant breast papillary lesions-B3 diagnosed on ultrasound-guided 14-gauge needle core biopsy: Analysis of 114 cases from a single institution and review of the literature. Pathol Oncol Res. 2015;21:535-546.

[33] Yamaguchi R, Tanaka M, Tse GM, Yamaguchi M, Terasaki H, Hirai Y, et al. Imaging-guided core needle biopsy of papillary lesions of the breast. Histopathology. 2015; 66(4):565-576

[34] Seely JM, Verma R, Kielar A, Smyth KR, Hack K, Taljaard M, Gravel D, Ellison E. Benign papillomas of the breast diagnosed on large-gauge vacuum biopsy compared with 14 gauge core needle biopsy – Do they require surgical excision? Breast J. 2017; 23(2):146-153.

[35] Fuentes JAP, Martínez CEM, Casadiego AKR, Freites VFA, Marín VAA, Castellano ACR. Papillary breast lesions diagnosed by percutaneous needle biopsy: Management approach. E Cancer Medical Science. 2019;13:902. DOI:10.3332/ecancer.2019.902

[36] Tokiniwa H, Horiguchi J, Takata D, et al. Papillary lesions of the breast diagnosed using core needle biopsies. Exp Ther Med. 2011;2(6):1069-1072. DOI:10.3892/etm.2011.332

[37] Ko ES, Cho N, Cha JH, Park JS, Kim SM, Moon WK. Sonographically-guided 14-gauge core needle biopsy for papillary lesions of the breast, if imaging findings also goes in favor. Korean J Radiol. 2007;8(3):206-211. DOI:10.3348/kjr.2007.8.3.206

[38] Rakha EA, Badve S, Eusebi V, et al. Breast lesions of uncertain malignant nature and limited metastatic potential: Proposals to improve their recognition and clinical management. Histopathology. 2016;68(1):45-56. DOI:10.1111/his.12861

Chapter 6

A Review of Progesterone Effects on Human Melanoma Cell Growth In-Vitro

Pandurangan Ramaraj

Abstract

Progesterone, a female sex hormone not only has a role in reproduction, but also in protecting females in melanoma. A survey of steroid hormones actions steroid hormones actions survey on melanoma cells and literature survey showed that progesterone inhibited mouse and human melanoma cell growth significantly in-vitro. Progesterone not only inhibited cell growth, but also affected adhesion and migration functions (essential for metastasis) in-vitro. This observation correlated with the clinical studies where they had shown showed an increased survival and delayed metastasis in menstruating females in melanoma. Further, progesterone level in menstruating females (1000–1500 ng/dL) compared to post-menopausal females (20–100 ng/dL) also correlated with previous clinical studies. Progesterone action on melanoma cells, as reported by other researchers also supported the findings from this lab. Hence, progesterone could be the steroid hormone protecting menstruating females in melanoma. Moreover, our recent studies showed that progesterone suppressed pro-inflammatory cytokine IL-8 secretion by the melanoma cells, which decreased melanoma cell growth in-vitro. Hence, progesterone apart from reproductive function may also be involved in protecting menstruating females in melanoma.

Keywords: progesterone, menstruating females, protection in melanoma, IL-8 secretion

1. Introduction

Skin is not only a largest organ in the body, but also an endocrine organ and a target site for other hormones [1–3]. Skin has all the elements of a functional hypothalamo-pituitary-adrenal axis [4]. So, it has CRH (corticotropic releasing hormone), POMC (pre-opiomelano cortin) and associated peptides ACTH (adreno corticotropic hormone), α-MSH (α-melanocyte stimulating hormone), β-endorphin [5]. Expression of these peptides is environmentally regulated and their dysfunction can lead to skin and systemic diseases [6]. Skin neuroendocrine system acts by preserving and maintaining the skin structural and functional integrity [7]. This network allow skin to maintain local and global homeostasis that is vital for survival [6, 7]. Skin and hair follicles not only have functional melatonin receptor, but to a larger extent serve as an extra-pineal organ to synthesize melatonin [8]. Skin has the ability to synthesize glucocorticoid from cholesterol or from steroid intermediates of systemic origin [6]. By interacting with glucocorticoid receptor, immune functions and physiological functions of epidermal, dermal and subcutaneous structures are regulated [9]. Since, synthesis and site of actions of hormones are nearby, it suggests auto, para and intracrine mode of actions. Levels of local production changes in response to environmental stress. This local glucosteroidogenesis is essential for skin homeostasis and prevent skin pathology. Sex steroids such as androgens, estrogens and progestins are essential for a healthy skin [1, 2]. Melanocyte, which is transformed to melanoma is also under the influence of melanocyte stimulating hormone (MSH) from pituitary. Generally, melanoma is not labeled as a hormone dependent cancer because of the fact that ultraviolet (UV) rays from the Sun is the major cause for melanoma [10]. UV rays cause deoxy ribonucleic acid (DNA) damages and other inflammatory changes in the skin, which result in skin cancer [11]. About 90% of melanoma is caused by environmental factors such as UV rays, radiations and only 10% is inherited in the family. So, melanoma is never considered as a hormone dependent cancer. However, existing evidences point to a hormone relatedness to survival or a hormone responsive nature of melanoma [12, 13].

2. In-vitro studies from our lab

In-vitro studies from our lab showed the involvement of progesterone in the regulation of mouse and human melanoma cell growth.

2.1 Effect of Steroids on mouse melanoma (B16F10) cell growth

Initially four sex steroids viz., dehydroepiandsterone (DHEA), androstenedione (AD), testosterone (T) and progesterone (P4) were used to find out their effect on mouse melanoma (B16F10) cell growth. Though all four steroids showed a dose-dependent decrease in cell growth, yet progesterone alone showed a significant inhibition of the mouse melanoma cell growth [14].

2.2 Dose-response curves with mouse (B16F10) and human (BLM) melanoma cells

As the initial study was carried out at high concentrations (100, 150 and 200 μM). dose-response study was carried out to rule out toxic effect of steroids on melanoma cell growth inhibition. Mouse (B16F10) and human melanoma (BLM) cells showed a dose-dependent cell growth inhibition, suggesting the inhibition was a biological action and not a toxic inhibition of cell growth at high concentrations [14, 15].

2.3 Effect of related steroids on mouse melanoma cell growth

A weak androgen DHEA also inhibited mouse melanoma cell growth, but it was not as significant as the inhibition of progesterone on mouse melanoma cells. But, RU-486 a progesterone receptor antagonist and also a glucocorticoid receptor antagonist showed significant inhibition of mouse melanoma cell growth [14, 15].

2.4 Mechanism of progesterone and RU-486 actions

Since progesterone and its receptor antagonist (RU-486) showed significant inhibition on melanoma cell growth, it raised the question whether progesterone receptor was involved in this action. However, a co-incubation experiment of progesterone and RU-486 showed an additive effect on melanoma cell growth inhibition, suggesting that the action was not mediated through progesterone receptor and that each hormone acted through different mechanisms resulting in an additive effect on the inhibition of melanoma cell growth. Similarly human melanoma cell growth showed an additive effect on cell growth inhibition, when progesterone at fixed concentration (10 μM) was co-incubated with varying concentrations of RU-486 (10, 50 and 100 μM).

2.5 Dose-curve with cholesterol to check non-specific action of steroids

Since inhibition was seen with DHEA, progesterone and RU-486, it raised the question whether it was a specific effect on melanoma cell lines or common effect on all cancer cell lines? So, cells were incubated with cholesterol the parent compound of all steroids. Though, cholesterol showed initial decrease in cell growth, it failed to show a dose-dependent inhibition of cell growth. It was almost flat line from 10 μM to 200 μM, suggesting that the inhibition by progesterone and RU-486 was specific to melanoma cells.

2.6 Effect of progesterone and RU-486 on human gastric cancer cell (NUGC3) line

The effect of progesterone and RU-486 seen on mouse and human melanoma cells raised the question whether it was a non-specific effect on melanoma cell lines. So, progesterone and RU-486 were incubated separately with human gastric cancer (NUGC3) cell line. Progesterone and RU-486 did not show a significant inhibition as seen that of on melanoma cells, suggesting the inhibition was specific to melanoma cells.

2.7 Effect of progesterone and RU-486 on normal rat vascular smooth muscle cells

So far experiments were carried out on transformed cells and hence the effect on normal cells was not known. So, normal rat vascular smooth muscle cells were used. Progesterone and RU-486 were incubated with smooth muscle cells, which did not show a significant inhibition, suggesting progesterone and RU-486 inhibition were specific to melanoma cells.

2.8 Mechanism of inhibition of human melanoma cell growth

As progesterone showed a dose-dependent inhibition of human melanoma (BLM) cell growth, the mechanism of inhibition was determined. After ruling out necrosis and apoptosis, autophagy [12] as the mechanism was detected by co-incubation with 3-MA (methyl adenine) and progesterone. Results showed a partial increase in cell growth (rescue of cell growth) with 3-MA and progesterone co-incubation compared to cells incubated with progesterone alone, suggesting the mechanism of inhibition of cell growth was due to autophagy.

2.9 Other in-vitro functions inhibited by progesterone

Progesterone not only inhibited cell growth, but also other in-vitro functions such as adhesion and migration. Both adhesion and migration functions were essential for metastasis. Clinical study showed that menstruating females were better protected in melanoma in terms of increased survival and delayed metastasis than post-menopausal women and men of any age. Literature survey also revealed that progesterone level in menstruating females was 100–150 ng/ml in the follicular phase and 1000–1500 ng/dL in the luteal phase [16]. Whereas, post-menopausal females' progesterone level was 20–100 ng/dL and males' levels were between 27 and 90 ng/dL. The last two groups were not protected in melanoma, as per the clinical studies. In fact, progesterone in-vitro action also suggested the same. Study of progesterone effect on melanoma cells by other researchers also showed the effect of progesterone on other human melanoma cell lines. Fang et al. from China showed inhibition of A375 and A875 cell line growth by progesterone and RU-486 and that their actions were not mediated through progesterone receptor [17]. Moroni et al. [18] repeated the study with the same lines using progesterone concentrations up to 1000 μM. Kanda and Watanbe [19] already showed the inhibition of human melanoma cell growth by progesterone along with dihydrotestosterone (DHT) and estradiol (E2). However, these studies did not correlate progesterone with the protective function as reported by the clinical studies.

3. Summary

Progesterone, a female sex steroid significantly inhibited mouse and human melanoma cell growth significantly in-vitro. RU-486, a progesterone receptor antagonist also significantly inhibited melanoma cell growth significantly. But the action was not mediated through progesterone receptor. In addition, effect of progesterone and RU-486 were found to be not a spurious or a toxic action. In-vitro studies also showed that progesterone inhibited human melanoma cells and the mechanism of inhibition was due to autophagy. Progesterone also inhibited adhesion and migration functions (essential for metastasis) of human melanoma cells in-vitro. This observation correlated well with the previous clinical studies which reported that menstruating females were better protected (increased survival and delayed metastasis) in melanoma than post-menopausal women and men of any age. Research works around the globe also showed inhibition of human melanoma cells by progesterone. Progesterone action was mediated by the suppression of IL-8 secretion by melanoma cells.

4. Conclusion

As shown by the in-vitro studies, progesterone could be protecting menstruating females in melanoma. In fact progesterone could be the appropriate steroid because progesterone is anti-inflammatory in nature. Further studies from our lab showed that progesterone suppressed pro-inflammatory cytokine IL-8 [20]. In fact, progesterone could be the appropriate steroid because progesterone is anti-inflammatory in nature. So, progesterone action could be mediated by the suppression of pro-inflammatory cytokine IL-8, which decreased melanoma cell growth in-vitro. Hence, survival of menstruating females in melanoma may be dependent on progesterone. So, progesterone apart from its effect on reproduction has also a role in protecting females from melanoma.

Author details

Pandurangan Ramaraj
Department of Biochemistry, Kirksville College of Osteopathic Medicine, A.T. Still University, Kirksville, MO, United States

*Address all correspondence to: pramaraj@atsu.edu

References

[1] Zouboulis CC, Chen WC, Thornton MJ, Qin K, Rosenfield R. Sexual hormones in human skin. Hormone and Metabolic Research. 2007;**39**(2):85-95

[2] Zouboulis CC. The human skin as a hormone target and an endocrine gland. Hormones. 2004;**3**(1):9-26

[3] Zouboulis CC. Human skin: An independent peripheral endocrine organ. Hormone Research. 2000; **54**:230-242

[4] Slominski A, Wortsman J. Neuroendocrinoloy of the skin. Endocrine Reviews. 2000;**21**(5):457-487

[5] Slominski A, Wortsman J. Self-regulated endocrine systems in the skin. Minerva Endocrinologica. 2003; **28**(2):135-143

[6] Slominski A, Zbytek B, Nikolakis G, Manna PR, Skobowiat C, Zmijewski M, et al. Steroidogenesis in the skin: Implications for local immune functions. The Journal of Steroid Biochemistry and Molecular Biology. 2013;**137**:107-123. DOI: 10.1016/j.jsbmb.2013.02.006. Epub 2013 Feb19

[7] Nikolakis G, Stratakis CA, Kanaki T, Slominski A, Zouboulis CC. Skin steroidogenesis in health and disease. Reviews in Endocrine & Metabolic Disorders. 2016;**17**(3):247-258

[8] Cos S, Garcia-Bolado A, Sanchez-Barcelo E. Direct antiproliferative effects of melatonin on two metastatic cell sub-lines of mouse melanoma (B16BL6 and PG19). Melanoma Research. 2001;**11**(2):197-201

[9] Labrie F. DHEA and its transformation into androgens and estrogens in peripheral target tissues: Intracrinology. Frontieres in Neuroendocrinology. 2001;**22**(3): 185-212

[10] Rass K, Reicharth J. UV damage and DNA repair in malignant melanoma and non-melanoma skin cancer. Advances in Experimental Medicine and Biology. 2008;**624**:162-178. DOI: 10.1007/978-0-387-77574-6_13

[11] Gray-Schopfer V, Wellbrock C, Marais R. Melanoma biology and new targeted therapy. Nature. 2007; **445**:851-857

[12] Ghosh R, Ott AM, Seetharam D, Slaga TJ, Kumar AP. Cell cycle block and apoptosis induction in a human melanoma cell line following treatment with 2-methoxyostradiol: Therapeutic implications? Melanoma Research. 2003;**13**(2):119-127

[13] Disorbo DM, McNulty B, Nathanson L. In vitro growth inhibition of human malignant melanoma cells by glucocorticoids. Cancer Research. 1983; **43**:2664-2667

[14] Ramaraj P, Cox JL. In-vitro effect of sex steroids on mouse melanoma (B16F10) cell growth. CellBio. 2014;**3**:60-71. DOI: 10.4236/cellbio.2014.32007

[15] Ramaraj P, Cox JL. In-vitro effect of progesterone on human melanoma (BLM) cell growth. International Journal of Clinical and Experimental Medicine. 2014;**7**(11):3941-3953

[16] Häggström M. Reference ranges for estradiol, progesterone, luteinizing hormone and follicle-stimulating hormone during the menstrual cycle. WikiJournal of Medicine. 2014;**1**(1):1. DOI: 10.15347/wjm/2014.001

[17] Fang X, Zhang X, Zhou M, Li J. Effects of progesterone on the growth regulation in classical progesterone

receptor-negative malignant melanoma cells. Journal of Huazhong University of Science and Technology Medical Sciences. 2010;**30**(2):231-234. DOI: 10.1007/s 11596-010-0220-3

[18] Moroni G, Gaziano R, Bue C, Agostini M, Perno CF, Sinibaldi-Vallebona P, et al. Progesterone and melanoma cells: An old story suspended between life and death. Journal of Steroids and Hormonal Science. 2015;**S13**:158. DOI: 10.4172/2157-7536.1000158

[19] Kanda N, Watanbe S. 17-β-estradiol, progesterone and dihydrotestosterone suppress the growth of human melanoma by inhibiting interleukin-8 production. The Journal of Investigative Dermatology. 2001;**117**:274-283

[20] Miller A, Fulcher A, Dock P, Ramaraj P. Biochemical basis of protection by progesterone in melanoma based on curcumin pre-treatment of human melanoma cell models. Endo2018Home. 2018. Available from: http://www.abstractsonline.com/pp8/#!/4482/presentation/7469

Section 4

Pathogenesis of Breast Cancer

Chapter 7

Regulation of Exosomes in the Pathogenesis of Breast Cancer

Congjian Shi, Hongqin Yang, Zhengchao Wang and Zhenghong Zhang

Abstract

Extracellular vesicles (EVs) are a heterogeneous group of endogenous nanoscale vesicles that are secreted by various cell types. Based on their biogenesis and size distribution, EVs can be broadly classified as exosomes and microvesicles. Exosomes are enveloped by lipid bilayers with a size of 30–150 nm in diameter, which contain diverse biomolecules, including lipids, proteins and nucleic acids. Exosomes transport their bioactive cargoes from original cells to recipient cells, thus play crucial roles in mediating intercellular communication. Breast cancer is the most common malignancy among women and remains a major health problem worldwide, diagnostic strategies and therapies aimed at breast cancer are still limited. Growing evidence shows that exosomes are involved in the pathogenesis of breast cancer, including tumorigenesis, invasion and metastasis. Here, we provide a straightforward overview of exosomes and highlight the role of exosomes in the pathogenesis of breast cancer, moreover, we discuss the potential application of exosomes as biomarkers and therapeutic tools in breast cancer diagnostics and therapeutics.

Keywords: extracellular vesicles, exosomes, breast cancer, miRNAs

1. Introduction

Extracellular vesicles (EVs) are heterogeneous membrane-bound vesicles which originate from endosomal or plasma membrane called exosomes or microvesicles, respectively [1]. The release of EVs was initially identified as a mode for cells to eliminate unwanted substances, however, the initial view with regard to EVs has changed dramatically with the deepening of research, and their crucial roles in diverse physiological and pathological processes have attracted extensive attention. According to their original cells, EVs are loaded with a specific set of preassembled bioactive cargoes, and give rise to phenotypic and genotypic changes in recipient cells [2, 3]. These cargoes enclosed within EVs are biologically significant, for example, three EV subtypes including one microvesicle and two exosome populations released by LIM1863 CRC (colorectal cancer) cells have distinct miRNA expression profiles [4]. EVs contribute to numerous aspects of normal physiological processes, including blood coagulation, immune surveillance, tissue repair and stem cell maintenance [5]. They are also closely related with diverse human diseases, including cancer, infectious diseases, neurologic diseases and cardiometabolic diseases [6]. Exosomes are a subtype of EVs and the application of exosomes as biomarkers

IntechOpen

and therapeutic tools has appeared as a promising area of research due to some preponderant properties of exosomes. Exosomes can be released according to the command received from adjacent and distant cells, or in response to the stimulation induced by local conditions [7]. Both normal and pathological cells are capable of secreting exosomes and they are stable in biological fluids [8]. Breast cancer is the most common malignancy affecting women, and its morbidity and mortality are estimated to increase in the coming years [9]. One in eight to ten women will be diagnosed with breast cancer during their lifetime [10], and breast cancer has seriously affected women's health. Accumulating evidence indicates that exosomes are involved in the pathogenesis of breast cancer, including tumorigenesis, invasion and metastasis. Studies focused on exosomes might provide novel perspectives for revealing breast cancer pathogenesis and improving the current poor diagnostic and therapeutic status of breast cancer.

2. Extracellular vesicles

Cells naturally release EVs into the extracellular space, these nanoscale vesicles encompassing bioactive cargoes play crucial roles in diverse physiological and pathological processes. The term EVs represent several subtypes of vesicles, standardized criteria for distinguishing EVs subtypes are still under discussion, but it is universally acknowledged that they can be classified as two main categories: exosomes and microvesicles. Other EVs subtypes such as apoptotic bodies [11], spheresomes [12] and large oncosomes [13], are not mentioned in this review. Exosomes have endosomal origin, they are 30–150 nm in diameter and float at a density of 1.13–1.19 g/ml in sucrose gradient [14, 15]. Exosomes are essentially intraluminal vesicles (ILVs) generated by inward budding of endosomal membrane during the maturation of endosomes, then released to the extracellular space when multivesicular bodies (MVBs) (also referred to late endosomes) fuse with plasma membranes [16, 17]. Microvesicles, typically larger than exosomes (100–1000 nm in diameter), arise through direct outward budding and fission of plasma membrane [18], hence, the membrane composition of microvesicles can better reflect the membrane composition of original cells in contrast to exosomes. Although the origin of exosomes and microvesicles occurs at distinct intracellular locations, some common mechanisms participate in both processes. The modes by which recipient cells take up EVs including endocytosis, direct membrane fusion and receptor ligand binding [19], but the specific molecular mechanisms deserve further investigation.

At present, the biogenesis of EVs, the substances they contain and the biological effects they promote have been extensively studied, which make people find out the potential of EVs in clinical application. EVs subtypes like exosomes and microvesicles may perform different functions, and it is absolutely necessary to isolate high-purity EVs subtypes, which will be crucial for EV-related functionality and therapeutic value studies. But even in EV preparations with high-purity, electron microscopy (EM) results imply that they still contain co-purifying elements [20]. The isolation of EVs is challenging because EVs subtypes have some similarities, including their size, density, composition, and surface marker proteins [21]. Meanwhile, EVs derived from biological fluids contain a mixture of multiple EVs secreted by various cell types [22]. Therefore, it is imperative to formulate universal standard protocols for the preparation of EVs.

Due to some peculiar characteristics of EVs, they have prominent biotechnological potential. EVs are biocompatible and safe, coupled with nanoscale diameter, resulting in their long blood circulation half-life and high drug loading capacity, which makes them possible to be ideal drug delivery vehicles [23]. EVs represent an attractive group of therapeutic biomarkers and has tremendous potential in immune response regulation and tissue regeneration [5, 24]. EVs are extensively found in diverse bodily fluids, and it is a promising area to serve EVs as biomarkers for early diagnosis and accurate prognosis. Since EVs are derived from bodily fluids, the diagnostic methods are probably non-invasive and considerably less painful than some existing diagnostic methods (for example, liver biopsy). Meanwhile, the clinical application of EVs can also monitor the response of therapy, which will contribute to convalescent process.

3. Exosomes

Exosomes are enveloped by lipid bilayers and act as mediators of intercellular communication through transmitting diverse functional biomolecules from original cells to recipient cells, and they are secreted by virtually all cell types, such as stem cells, immune cells and tumor cells [25]. The cargoes transported by exosomes including lipids, proteins, RNA (coding and non-coding) and even DNA (genomic and mitochondrial) [26]. Exosomes can be detected and isolated from diverse bodily fluids, exemplified by blood, urine, saliva, cerebrospinal fluid and breast milk [27], they can also be obtained from cell culture-conditioned media [28]. Some specific surface proteins are considered as the makers of exosome, such as tetraspanin family (CD9, CD63 and CD81), heat shock protein 70 (HSP70) and major histocompatibility complex (MHC) molecules [29]. Exosomes also contain abundant ceramide, cholesterol and sphingomyelin, which may relate to their lipid raft microdomains [30]. Multiple genetic materials are detected in exosomes, and exosome-encapsulated miRNAs have obtained extra attention because of their vital roles in regulating gene expression and can be used as biomarkers for a variety of diseases [31].

Exosomes exhibit unique biogenesis mechanism. Plasma membrane buds inward through endocytosis, resulting the generation of early endosomes [32]. The process from early endosomes to late endosomes (also referred to MVBs) requires the involvement of Golgi complex, during which ILVs also accumulate by the invagination of endosomal membrane in their lumen [15]. Then, MVBs either fuse with lysosomes, which ILVs are degraded, or fuse with plasma membranes, which ILVs are released to the extracellular space as exosomes [33]. Fusion of MVBs with plasma membrane requires the assistance of soluble N-ethylmaleimide-sensitive fusion attachment protein receptor (SNARE) complexes [34]. The endosomal sorting complex required for transport (ESCRT) machinery, a vital participant in exosome biogenesis, is responsible for ILVs formation and protein sorting [35]. ESCRT machinery contains four complexes, ESCRT-0, ESCRT-I, ESCRT-II and ESCRT-III, as well as associated proteins, including ALIX, VPS4 and VTA1 [36]. ESCRT-0 recognizes the ubiquitinated cargoes, ESCRT-I and ESCRT-II initiate the budding process of ILVs, whereas ESCRT-III terminates this process [3, 37]. ESCRT-independent mechanisms also exist by the evidence that MVBs still form in the absence of ESCRTs [38], further studies report that the mechanisms are related with the sphingolipid ceramide [39] or some members of the tetraspanin family [40]. In single MVBs, a competitive relationship between ESCRT-dependent and ESCRT-independent mechanisms exists, which affects the size of ILVs formed inside [41], this makes it possible to identify different subpopulations of MVBs based on their ILVs size. A group of Rab GTPases including Rab11, Rab27a, and Rab27b, are also involved in the release of exosomes [42]. Once exosomes are released to the extracellular space, they may exist in the circulation or be taken up by adjacent and distant cells [43, 44].

Exosomal preparations with high-purity are significant for further exploration of exosomal biogenesis and functions, and techniques for exosomal isolation have made great advances. At present, the commonly used isolation techniques including ultracentrifugation-based techniques, size-based techniques, precipitation, immunocapture and microfluidic-based techniques [35, 45] (**Table 1**). Among them, ultracentrifugation is the most extensively used exosomal isolation technique for bodily fluids and cell culture supernatant [46]. Each technique has its own merits and demerits, and the combination of aforementioned techniques may lead to a more desirable isolation. Recent study showed that the acidic condition was more suitable for the isolation of exosomes [47], indicating that local pH of exosomes should be taken into account for future researches.

Specific roles of the tumor microenvironment during cancer progression and metastasis have been widely studied [48], and cancer cell–derived exosomes can establish a favorable microenvironment to induce cell proliferation, angiogenesis, resistance to apoptosis and initiation of pre-metastatic niches through their bioactive content [22, 49]. The secretion of exosome appears to have an impact on drug resistance, for example, exosomes enriched in TAG72 imply that CRC patients might be resistant to 5-FU [50]. And cells under pathological status release even more exosomes, it is estimated that there are approximately 2,000 trillion exosomes presented in normal human blood and 4,000 trillion exosomes presented in the blood of cancer patients [51]. According to these results, it is feasible to serve exosomes as biomarkers for diagnosis and prognosis. Exosomes are capable of inducing anti-tumor responses through delivering tumor antigens to immune cells, and exosomes derived from T cells can suppress tumor development [52], demonstrating their great potential in modulating immune responses. Enlightened by the capability of exosomes that transmits biomolecules from original cells to recipient cells, accompanied with their biocompatibility, low immunogenicity and toxicity, high stability in the circulation, biological barrier permeability and potential targeting to specific sites [53], diverse strategies have been developed for loading therapeutic cargoes into exosomes, which have a broad application prospect.

Exosome plays important roles in tumor diagnostics and therapeutics. Tissue biopsy is usually acquired from the site of primary tumor and reflects its molecular traits over a period of time, therapies will be determined according to the results of tissue biopsy. However, the limitations of tissue biopsy are obvious, it is not comprehensive enough to reflect heterogeneity and dynamic evolution of tumor [54].

Isolation techniques	Advantages	Disadvantages	References
Ultracentrifugation-based techniques	Low cost, most commonly used	Time-consuming, high equipment cost, low recovery	[15, 45]
Size-based techniques	Fast, convenient, high yield	Lack specificity, requires dedicated equipment	[17, 46]
Precipitation	Easy, does not require specialized equipment	Lack specificity, time-consuming	[15, 45, 46]
Immunocapture	High purity	Expensive, low capacity	[28, 35]
Microfluidic-based techniques	Fast, low cost, convenient	Lack standardization and large-scale tests on clinical samples, lack method validation	[45, 52]

Table 1.
The advantages and disadvantages of different techniques used for exosome isolation.

Exosome related liquid biopsy techniques including surface-enhanced Raman spectroscopy (SERS), next generation sequencing (NGS), digital droplet PCR (ddPCR) and molecular barcoding, have drawn extra attention due to its unique advantages of minimally invasive and serial biochemical tests [55]. Among diversified methods developed for liquid biopsy, SERS-based technique for detection of circulating tumor markers including exosomes is one of the most powerful methods, it owns the advantages of high sensitivity, specificity, tremendous spectral multiplexing capacity for simultaneous target detection, and its unique capability for obtaining intrinsic fingerprint spectra of biomolecules [56]. The application of exosome related liquid biopsy enables the improvement of various aspects of tumor management including early diagnosis and screening, prediction of prognosis, early detection of relapse, serial sampling and efficient longitudinal monitoring of disease progress and response to treatment [57]. Although exosome related liquid biopsy is a promising area, there are still some loopholes including difficult extraction and did not analyze the phenotypic studies of cells from tumor, that require further refinement and validation [58].

4. Breast cancer

Breast cancer is a disease with high heterogeneity, containing multiple tumor entities that have diverse clinical behavior and biological features [59], which complicate its diagnosis and treatment. Among women, breast cancer is the most common malignancy and the second leading causes of cancer-related death [60]. The 5-year overall survival rate for non-metastatic breast cancer patients is greater than 80%, whereas distant metastasis can reduce this rate to approximately 25%, and the main metastatic sites including bone, brain, liver and lung [61]. The diagnosis and treatment of patients are evaluated by clinical assessment, breast imaging, tumor size, histologic grade, lymph node involvement or acknowledged biomarkers, including estrogen receptor (ER), human epidermal growth factor receptor 2 (HER2) and progesterone receptor (PR) [62]. The clinical classification of breast cancer should be reasonable, so as to select the most appropriate diagnostic strategy and therapy for each patient, and the molecular subtypes of breast cancer are represented by basal-like, HER2-enriched, normal breast-like, luminal A, luminal B and claudin-low [63]. The occurrence of breast cancer is influenced by age, race, obesity, smoke, drinking, oral contraceptives and other exogenous estrogens, age at menarche, age at menopause, age at first live birth and environmental toxins [64, 65], also, inherited genetic mutations are responsible for 5–10% of all breast cancer cases, and mutations in BRCA1 and BRCA2 are believed to increase the lifetime risk of being diagnosed with breast cancer by more than four times [66].

Breast cancer is generally diagnosed by mammography, computed tomography (CT), magnetic resonance imaging (MRI), ultrasound, core needle biopsy, excisional biopsy and histopathologic evaluation [65, 67]. Diagnosed patients with parallel clinical and biological characteristics may exhibit distinct responses to treatment and bring about different outcomes [68], therefore, the research on breast cancer treatment needs to be further deepened. At present, surgery and radiation are mentioned frequently in treatment, and three approaches are primarily adopted in medical oncology: ER + -related breast cancer aimed at anti-endocrine strategies, HER2 + -related breast cancer treated with HER2-targeted drugs and triple-negative breast cancer (TNBC) managed with traditional cytotoxic therapy [69]. More importantly, it is not just about choosing the appropriate treatment for each patient, the sequencing of therapies should also be considered.

5. Exosomal functionality and therapeutic value in breast cancer

It has been widely acknowledged that exosomes are important players in the pathogenesis of breast cancer (**Figure 1**). The release of exosomes induced by heparanase, hypoxia and other stimulation is involved in breast cancer angiogenesis, which facilitate tumorigenesis process of breast cancer [70]. Also, exosomes promote breast cancer tumorigenesis by modifying tumor microenvironment to permissive niches. Typically, alteration in miRNAs expression have been found to influence initiation and development of breast cancer [71], for example, compared with non-malignant breast cells or non-metastatic breast cancer cells, exosomal miR-10b is significantly upregulated in metastatic breast cancer cells [72]. Further research shows that RNA induced silencing complex-loading complex (RLC) proteins Dicer, AGO2 and TRBP, which have been proved to participate in miRNA biogenesis, can be detected in exosomes derived from the serum of breast cancer patients and breast cancer cells, moreover, Dicer inhibition in cancer exosomes obviously decelerates tumor growth in recipient cells [73]. Invasion plays an important role in cancer development, invasion ability of non-malignant breast cells can be induced by exosomes derived from metastatic breast cancer cells [72]. Metastatic breast cancer cells specifically express and release miR-105, during which exosomal miR-105 can transfer to endothelial cells and acts as an effective regulator of their migration [74]. Recent study also suggested that miR-7641 was identified as an important component of exosomes that could promote breast tumor metastasis [75]. Drug resistance are also closely related with exosomes as they are capable of transporting anti-cancer drugs outside breast cancer cells. Chen et al. reported that drug-resistant breast cancer cells might spread their drug-resistant capacity to sensitive cells through secreting exosomes, they further confirmed that this

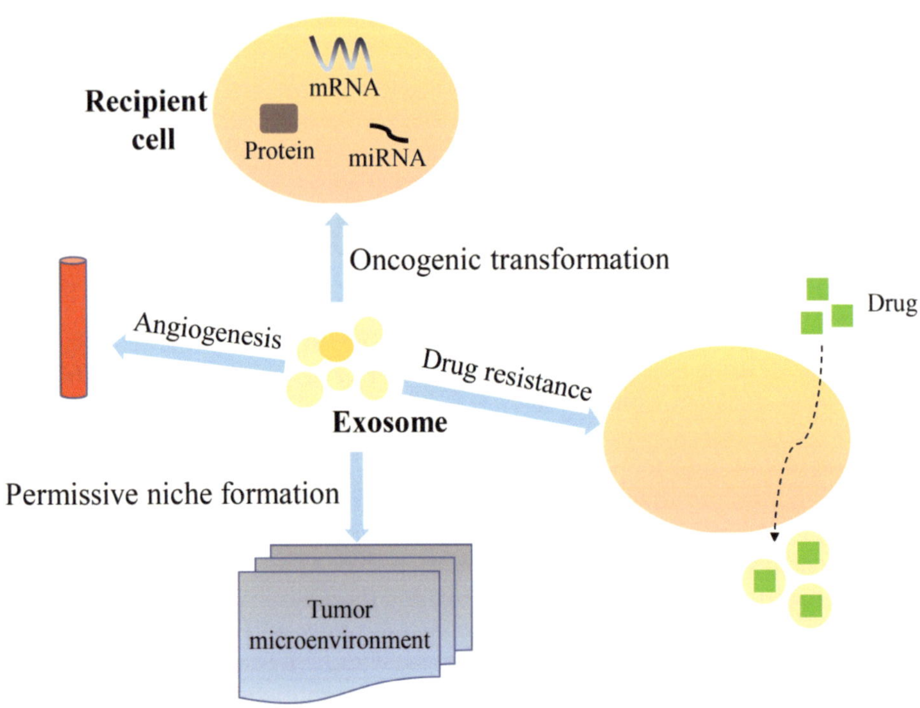

Figure 1.
Exosome in the pathogenesis of breast cancer. Exosome contribute to oncogenic transformation, angiogenesis, permissive niche formation and drug resistance in breast cancer.

process was mediated by exosomal miRNAs [76]. Trastuzumab is a commonly used drugs to treat breast cancer, while exosome-transmitted cicHIPK3 could promote trastuzumab chemoresistance of drug-sensitive BC cells, decreasing the therapeutic effect [77]. Recent study showed that exosomal miR-155 regulated drug resistance of breast cancer [78] and chemotherapy with miR-155-targeting therapies may lead to satisfactory outcomes.

Breast cancer is a disease which tends to metastasis, patients with early diagnosis, reasonable prognosis and accurate treatment usually have more favorable outcomes, yet approaches against breast cancer are still limited, and exosomes could be employed as novel biomarkers and therapeutic tools for patients with breast cancer. Hannafon and colleagues found that exosomes derived from breast cancer cells were enriched with specific miRNAs (miR-1246 and miR-21), what's more, these miRNAs in plasma exosomes of breast cancer patients were significantly higher than those of healthy control subjects [79], and exosomes may play crucial roles as biomarkers for breast cancer. Distant metastasis or local recurrence of breast cancer are strongly related with exosomal miRNAs, including miR-17-5p, miR-93-5p, miR-130a-3p, miR-340-5p [80], which can serve as indicators for prognosis. Now that exosomes remain stable in biological fluids, they are also promising for early diagnosis or monitoring the treatment process of breast cancer. In contrast to delivering anticancer drugs outside breast cancer cells, exosomes can also target anticancer drugs to breast cancer cells after appropriate modifications, for example, exosomes modified by targeting ligands deliver doxorubicin to tumors [81], which improve the therapeutic efficacy. Exosomes derived from mesenchymal stem cells (MSCs) can be used as drug delivery vehicles to transport locked nucleic acid (LNA)-anti-miR-142-3p, therefore reducing tumorigenicity in breast cancer [82].

6. Summary

Over the past few decades, on account of great advances in our understanding of breast cancer biology, diverse diagnostic and prognostic strategies, as well as targeted therapies are continuously evolving, while the situation of breast cancer patients remains unsatisfactory. For prevention and treatment of breast cancer, we need not only to develop new biomarkers and therapeutic tools, but also to further investigate the potential molecular mechanisms. Fortunately, accompany by our comprehension of exosomes is becoming more refined, the role of exosomes in initiation and development of breast cancer has been widely explored, and it is meaningful to translate exosomal research achievements to develop safe and effective therapies, diagnostic methods, along with drug delivery vehicles, which may conduce to improve the unsatisfactory situation of breast cancer patients.

Acknowledgements

This study was supported by the Special Funds of the Central Government Guiding Local Science and Technology Development (2020L3008), Provincial Natural Science Foundation (2018J01721, 2018J01721, 2019J01674 and 2020J01176), the Educational Reform Project (Y201809 and I202003009) and Training Program of Innovation and Entrepreneurship for Undergraduates (CXXL2020291 and CXXL2020293) of the Fujian Normal University.

Author details

Congjian Shi, Hongqin Yang, Zhengchao Wang and Zhenghong Zhang*
Provincial Key Laboratory for Developmental Biology and Neurosciences, Key Laboratory of Optoelectronic Science and Technology for Medicine of Ministry of Education, College of Life Sciences, Fujian Normal University, Fuzhou, China

*Address all correspondence to: zhangzh@fjnu.edu.cn

References

[1] G. van Niel, G. D'Angelo, G. Raposo, Shedding light on the cell biology of extracellular vesicles, Nat Rev Mol Cell Biol 19(4) (2018) 213-228.

[2] K.C. French, M.A. Antonyak, R.A. Cerione, Extracellular vesicle docking at the cellular port: Extracellular vesicle binding and uptake, Semin Cell Dev Biol 67 (2017) 48-55.

[3] C. D'Souza-Schorey, J.S. Schorey, Regulation and mechanisms of extracellular vesicle biogenesis and secretion, Essays Biochem 62(2) (2018) 125-133.

[4] H. Ji, M. Chen, D.W. Greening, W. He, A. Rai, W. Zhang, R.J. Simpson, Deep sequencing of RNA from three different extracellular vesicle (EV) subtypes released from the human LIM1863 colon cancer cell line uncovers distinct miRNA-enrichment signatures, PLoS One 9(10) (2014) e110314.

[5] E.L.A. S, I. Mager, X.O. Breakefield, M.J. Wood, Extracellular vesicles: biology and emerging therapeutic opportunities, Nat Rev Drug Discov 12(5) (2013) 347-357.

[6] R. Shah, T. Patel, J.E. Freedman, Circulating Extracellular Vesicles in Human Disease, N Engl J Med 379(10) (2018) 958-966.

[7] M.D. Mitchell, H.N. Peiris, M. Kobayashi, Y.Q. Koh, G. Duncombe, S.E. Illanes, G.E. Rice, C. Salomon, Placental exosomes in normal and complicated pregnancy, Am J Obstet Gynecol 213(4 Suppl) (2015) S173-S181.

[8] H. Im, K. Lee, R. Weissleder, H. Lee, C.M. Castro, Novel nanosensing technologies for exosome detection and profiling, Lab Chip 17(17) (2017) 2892-2898.

[9] Z. Anastasiadi, G.D. Lianos, E. Ignatiadou, H.V. Harissis, M. Mitsis, Breast cancer in young women: an overview, Updates Surg 69(3) (2017) 313-317.

[10] N. Harbeck, M. Gnant, Breast cancer, Lancet 389(10074) (2017) 1134-1150.

[11] X. Xu, Y. Lai, Z.C. Hua, Apoptosis and apoptotic body: disease message and therapeutic target potentials, Biosci Rep 39(1) (2019) BSR20180992.

[12] C. Junquera, T. Castiella, G. Munoz, R. Fernandez-Pacheco, M.J. Luesma, M. Monzon, Biogenesis of a new type of extracellular vesicles in gastrointestinal stromal tumors: ultrastructural profiles of spheresomes, Histochem Cell Biol 146(5) (2016) 557-567.

[13] V.R. Minciacchi, M.R. Freeman, D. Di Vizio, Extracellular vesicles in cancer: exosomes, microvesicles and the emerging role of large oncosomes, Semin Cell Dev Biol 40 (2015) 41-51.

[14] M.L. Merchant, I.M. Rood, J.K.J. Deegens, J.B. Klein, Isolation and characterization of urinary extracellular vesicles: implications for biomarker discovery, Nat Rev Nephrol 13(12) (2017) 731-749.

[15] C. He, S. Zheng, Y. Luo, B. Wang, Exosome Theranostics: Biology and Translational Medicine, Theranostics 8(1) (2018) 237-255.

[16] D.W. Greening, R. Xu, S.K. Gopal, A. Rai, R.J. Simpson, Proteomic insights into extracellular vesicle biology - defining exosomes and shed microvesicles, Expert Rev Proteomics 14(1) (2017) 69-95.

[17] H. Bu, D. He, X. He, K. Wang, Exosomes: Isolation, Analysis, and Applications in Cancer Detection and Therapy, Chembiochem 20(4) (2019) 451-461.

[18] L. Han, J. Xu, Q. Xu, B. Zhang, E.W. Lam, Y. Sun, Extracellular vesicles in the tumor microenvironment: Therapeutic resistance, clinical biomarkers, and targeting strategies, Med Res Rev 37(6) (2017) 1318-1349.

[19] H.K. Karnati, J.H. Garcia, D. Tweedie, R.E. Becker, D. Kapogiannis, N.H. Greig, Neuronal Enriched Extracellular Vesicle Proteins as Biomarkers for Traumatic Brain Injury, J Neurotrauma 36(7) (2019) 975-987.

[20] M. Gimona, K. Pachler, S. Laner-Plamberger, K. Schallmoser, E. Rohde, Manufacturing of Human Extracellular Vesicle-Based Therapeutics for Clinical Use, Int J Mol Sci 18(6) (2017) 1190.

[21] D.W. Greening, R.J. Simpson, Understanding extracellular vesicle diversity - current status, Expert Rev Proteomics 15(11) (2018) 887-910.

[22] C. Villarroya-Beltri, F. Baixauli, C. Gutierrez-Vazquez, F. Sanchez-Madrid, M. Mittelbrunn, Sorting it out: regulation of exosome loading, Semin Cancer Biol 28 (2014) 3-13.

[23] O.Y. Kim, J. Lee, Y.S. Gho, Extracellular vesicle mimetics: Novel alternatives to extracellular vesicle-based theranostics, drug delivery, and vaccines, Semin Cell Dev Biol 67 (2017) 74-82.

[24] S. Keshtkar, N. Azarpira, M.H. Ghahremani, Mesenchymal stem cell-derived extracellular vesicles: novel frontiers in regenerative medicine, Stem Cell Res Ther 9(1) (2018) 63.

[25] S. Cui, Z. Cheng, W. Qin, L. Jiang, Exosomes as a liquid biopsy for lung cancer, Lung Cancer 116 (2018) 46-54.

[26] S. Lakshmi, T.A. Hughes, S. Priya, Exosomes and exosomal RNAs in breast cancer: A status update, Eur J Cancer 144 (2020) 252-268.

[27] Y.F. Zhang, J.B. Shi, C. Li, Small extracellular vesicle loading systems in cancer therapy: Current status and the way forward, Cytotherapy 21(11) (2019) 1122-1136.

[28] K.W. Witwer, E.I. Buzas, L.T. Bemis, A. Bora, C. Lasser, J. Lotvall, E.N. Nolte-'t Hoen, M.G. Piper, S. Sivaraman, J. Skog, C. Thery, M.H. Wauben, F. Hochberg, Standardization of sample collection, isolation and analysis methods in extracellular vesicle research, J Extracell Vesicles 2 (2013) 20360.

[29] S. Lee, S. Mankhong, J.H. Kang, Extracellular Vesicle as a Source of Alzheimer's Biomarkers: Opportunities and Challenges, Int J Mol Sci 20(7) (2019) 1728.

[30] A.J. O'Loughlin, C.A. Woffindale, M.J. Wood, Exosomes and the emerging field of exosome-based gene therapy, Curr Gene Ther 12(4) (2012) 262-274.

[31] A. Thind, C. Wilson, Exosomal miRNAs as cancer biomarkers and therapeutic targets, J Extracell Vesicles 5 (2016) 31292.

[32] X. Xia, Y. Wang, Y. Huang, H. Zhang, H. Lu, J.C. Zheng, Exosomal miRNAs in central nervous system diseases: biomarkers, pathological mediators, protective factors and therapeutic agents, Prog Neurobiol 183 (2019) 101694.

[33] M. Klingeborn, W.M. Dismuke, C. Bowes Rickman, W.D. Stamer, Roles of exosomes in the normal and diseased eye, Prog Retin Eye Res 59 (2017) 158-177.

[34] M. Mathieu, L. Martin-Jaular, G. Lavieu, C. Thery, Specificities of secretion and uptake of exosomes and other extracellular vesicles for cell-to-cell communication, Nat Cell Biol 21(1) (2019) 9-17.

[35] E. Willms, C. Cabanas, I. Mager, M.J.A. Wood, P. Vader, Extracellular Vesicle Heterogeneity: Subpopulations, Isolation Techniques, and Diverse Functions in Cancer Progression, Front Immunol 9 (2018) 738.

[36] W.M. Henne, N.J. Buchkovich, S.D. Emr, The ESCRT pathway, Dev Cell 21(1) (2011) 77-91.

[37] D.S. Choi, D.K. Kim, Y.K. Kim, Y.S. Gho, Proteomics of extracellular vesicles: Exosomes and ectosomes, Mass Spectrom Rev 34(4) (2015) 474-490.

[38] S. Stuffers, C. Sem Wegner, H. Stenmark, A. Brech, Multivesicular endosome biogenesis in the absence of ESCRTs, Traffic 10(7) (2009) 925-937.

[39] K. Trajkovic, C. Hsu, S. Chiantia, L. Rajendran, D. Wenzel, F. Wieland, P. Schwille, B. Brugger, M. Simons, Ceramide triggers budding of exosome vesicles into multivesicular endosomes, Science 319(5867) (2008) 1244-1247.

[40] Z. Andreu, M. Yanez-Mo, Tetraspanins in extracellular vesicle formation and function, Front Immunol 5 (2014) 442.

[41] J.R. Edgar, E.R. Eden, C.E. Futter, Hrs- and CD63-dependent competing mechanisms make different sized endosomal intraluminal vesicles, Traffic 15(2) (2014) 197-211.

[42] E. de la Torre-Escudero, A.P.S. Bennett, A. Clarke, G.P. Brennan, M.W. Robinson, Extracellular Vesicle Biogenesis in Helminths: More than One Route to the Surface?, Trends Parasitol 32(12) (2016) 921-929.

[43] T. Vagner, A. Chin, J. Mariscal, S. Bannykh, D.M. Engman, D. Di Vizio, Protein Composition Reflects Extracellular Vesicle Heterogeneity, Proteomics 19(8) (2019) e1800167.

[44] A.M. Deleo, T. Ikezu, Extracellular Vesicle Biology in Alzheimer's Disease and Related Tauopathy, J Neuroimmune Pharm 13(3) (2018) 292-308.

[45] P. Li, M. Kaslan, S.H. Lee, J. Yao, Z. Gao, Progress in Exosome Isolation Techniques, Theranostics 7(3) (2017) 789-804.

[46] B.Y. Chen, C.W. Sung, C. Chen, C.M. Cheng, D.P. Lin, C.T. Huang, M.Y. Hsu, Advances in exosomes technology, Clin Chim Acta 493 (2019) 14-19.

[47] J.J. Ban, M. Lee, W. Im, M. Kim, Low pH increases the yield of exosome isolation, Biochem Biophys Res Commun 461(1) (2015) 76-79.

[48] D.F. Quail, J.A. Joyce, Microenvironmental regulation of tumor progression and metastasis, Nat Med 19(11) (2013) 1423-1437.

[49] S.W. Ferguson, J. Nguyen, Exosomes as therapeutics: The implications of molecular composition and exosomal heterogeneity, J Control Release 228 (2016) 179-190.

[50] Y. Xiao, Y. Li, Y. Yuan, B. Liu, S. Pan, Q. Liu, X. Qi, H. Zhou, W. Dong, L. Jia, The potential of exosomes derived from colorectal cancer as a biomarker, Clin Chim Acta 490 (2019) 186-193.

[51] R. Kalluri, The biology and function of exosomes in cancer, J Clin Invest 126(4) (2016) 1208-1215.

[52] E.V. Batrakova, M.S. Kim, Using exosomes, naturally-equipped nanocarriers, for drug delivery, J Control Release 219 (2015) 396-405.

[53] J. Meldolesi, Exosomes and Ectosomes in Intercellular Communication, Curr Biol 28(8) (2018) R435-R444.

[54] S. Mader, K. Pantel, Liquid Biopsy: Current Status and Future Perspectives,

Oncol Res Treat 40(7-8) (2017) 404-408.

[55] S. Alimirzaie, M. Bagherzadeh, M.R. Akbari, Liquid biopsy in breast cancer: A comprehensive review, Clin Genet 95(6) (2019) 643-660.

[56] Y. Zhang, X. Mi, X. Tan, R. Xiang, Recent Progress on Liquid Biopsy Analysis using Surface-Enhanced Raman Spectroscopy, Theranostics 9(2) (2019) 491-525.

[57] L. Giannopoulou, M. Zavridou, S. Kasimir-Bauer, E.S. Lianidou, Liquid biopsy in ovarian cancer: the potential of circulating miRNAs and exosomes, Transl Res 205 (2019) 77-91.

[58] J. Wang, S. Chang, G. Li, Y. Sun, Application of liquid biopsy in precision medicine: opportunities and challenges, Front Med 11(4) (2017) 522-527.

[59] B. Weigelt, J.S. Reis-Filho, Histological and molecular types of breast cancer: is there a unifying taxonomy?, Nat Rev Clin Oncol 6(12) (2009) 718-730.

[60] I. Januskeviciene, V. Petrikaite, Heterogeneity of breast cancer: The importance of interaction between different tumor cell populations, Life Sci 239 (2019) 117009.

[61] Y. Liang, H. Zhang, X. Song, Q. Yang, Metastatic heterogeneity of breast cancer: Molecular mechanism and potential therapeutic targets, Semin Cancer Biol 60 (2020) 14-27.

[62] M. Keshtgar, T. Davidson, K. Pigott, M. Falzon, A. Jones, Current status and advances in management of early breast cancer, Int J Surg 8(3) (2010) 199-202.

[63] P. Eroles, A. Bosch, J.A. Perez-Fidalgo, A. Lluch, Molecular biology in breast cancer: intrinsic subtypes and signaling pathways, Cancer Treat Rev 38(6) (2012) 698-707.

[64] G. Wong, E. Au, S.V. Badve, W.H. Lim, Breast Cancer and Transplantation, Am J Transplant 17(9) (2017) 2243-2253.

[65] C.B. Matsen, L.A. Neumayer, Breast cancer: a review for the general surgeon, JAMA Surg 148(10) (2013) 971-979.

[66] J.A. de la Mare, L. Contu, M.C. Hunter, B. Moyo, J.N. Sterrenberg, K.C. Dhanani, L.Z. Mutsvunguma, A.L. Edkins, Breast cancer: current developments in molecular approaches to diagnosis and treatment, Recent Pat Anticancer Drug Discov 9(2) (2014) 153-175.

[67] E.S. McDonald, A.S. Clark, J. Tchou, P. Zhang, G.M. Freedman, Clinical Diagnosis and Management of Breast Cancer, J Nucl Med 57 Suppl 1 (2016) 9S–16S.

[68] E.A. Rakha, M.E. El-Sayed, J.S. Reis-Filho, I.O. Ellis, Expression profiling technology: its contribution to our understanding of breast cancer, Histopathology 52(1) (2008) 67-81.

[69] K.A. Cadoo, T.A. Traina, T.A. King, Advances in molecular and clinical subtyping of breast cancer and their implications for therapy, Surg Oncol Clin N Am 22(4) (2013) 823-840.

[70] D.D. Yu, Y. Wu, H.Y. Shen, M.M. Lv, W.X. Chen, X.H. Zhang, S.L. Zhong, J.H. Tang, J.H. Zhao, Exosomes in development, metastasis and drug resistance of breast cancer, Cancer Sci 106(8) (2015) 959-964.

[71] S.H. Jafari, Z. Saadatpour, A. Salmaninejad, F. Momeni, M. Mokhtari, J.S. Nahand, M. Rahmati, H. Mirzaei, M. Kianmehr, Breast cancer diagnosis: Imaging techniques and biochemical markers, J Cell Physiol 233(7) (2018) 5200-5213.

[72] R. Singh, R. Pochampally, K. Watabe, Z. Lu, Y.Y. Mo,

Exosome-mediated transfer of miR-10b promotes cell invasion in breast cancer, Mol Cancer 13 (2014) 256.

[73] S.A. Melo, H. Sugimoto, J.T. O'Connell, N. Kato, A. Villanueva, A. Vidal, L. Qiu, E. Vitkin, L.T. Perelman, C.A. Melo, A. Lucci, C. Ivan, G.A. Calin, R. Kalluri, Cancer exosomes perform cell-independent microRNA biogenesis and promote tumorigenesis, Cancer Cell 26(5) (2014) 707-721.

[74] W. Zhou, M.Y. Fong, Y. Min, G. Somlo, L. Liu, M.R. Palomares, Y. Yu, A. Chow, S.T. O'Connor, A.R. Chin, Y. Yen, Y. Wang, E.G. Marcusson, P. Chu, J. Wu, X. Wu, A.X. Li, Z. Li, H. Gao, X. Ren, M.P. Boldin, P.C. Lin, S.E. Wang, Cancer-secreted miR-105 destroys vascular endothelial barriers to promote metastasis, Cancer Cell 25(4) (2014) 501-515.

[75] S. Shen, Y. Song, B. Zhao, Y. Xu, X. Ren, Y. Zhou, Q. Sun, Cancer-derived exosomal miR-7641 promotes breast cancer progression and metastasis, Cell Commun Signal 19(1) (2021) 20.

[76] C.Y. Wu, S.L. Du, J. Zhang, A.L. Liang, Y.J. Liu, Exosomes and breast cancer: a comprehensive review of novel therapeutic strategies from diagnosis to treatment, Cancer Gene Ther 24(1) (2017) 6-12.

[77] H. Zhang, C. Yan, Y. Wang, Exosome-mediated transfer of circHIPK3 promotes trastuzumab chemoresistance in breast cancer, J Drug Target (2021) 1-39.

[78] J.C. Santos, N.D.S. Lima, L.O. Sarian, A. Matheu, M.L. Ribeiro, S.F.M. Derchain, Exosome-mediated breast cancer chemoresistance via miR-155 transfer, Sci Rep 8(1) (2018) 829.

[79] B.N. Hannafon, Y.D. Trigoso, C.L. Calloway, Y.D. Zhao, D.H. Lum, A.L. Welm, Z.J. Zhao, K.E. Blick, W.C. Dooley, W.Q. Ding, Plasma exosome microRNAs are indicative of breast cancer, Breast Cancer Res 18(1) (2016) 90.

[80] M. Wang, S. Ji, G. Shao, J. Zhang, K. Zhao, Z. Wang, A. Wu, Effect of exosome biomarkers for diagnosis and prognosis of breast cancer patients, Clin Transl Oncol 20(7) (2018) 906-911.

[81] Y. Tian, S. Li, J. Song, T. Ji, M. Zhu, G.J. Anderson, J. Wei, G. Nie, A doxorubicin delivery platform using engineered natural membrane vesicle exosomes for targeted tumor therapy, Biomaterials 35(7) (2014) 2383-2390.

[82] Z. Naseri, R.K. Oskuee, M.R. Jaafari, M. Forouzandeh Moghadam, Exosome-mediated delivery of functionally active miRNA-142-3p inhibitor reduces tumorigenicity of breast cancer in vitro and in vivo, Int J Nanomedicine 13 (2018) 7727-7747.

Chapter 8

Long-Term Survivors of Breast Cancer: A Growing Population

Nadeem Bilani, Elizabeth Blessing Elimimian, Leah Elson, Hong Liang and Zeina Nahleh

Abstract

Breast cancer represents the most common malignancy among women. However, due to effective public health campaigns and updated screening guidelines, the annual incidence of late stage diagnoses has fallen. This stage migration has allowed for better prognosis and more women achieving long-term survival. In this chapter, we review long-term survivorship – defined as 10 years from diagnosis – as reported in the United States and around the world. Additionally, we provide analysis for socio-demographic, clinical and pathologic factors associated with 10-year survival, using data from a large national registry. This chapter also utilizes historical case data to forecast stage migration patterns in breast cancer diagnoses, within the United States, to 2030. Finally, we discuss the effects of the novel coronavirus pandemic on breast cancer treatment and access to care, with a review of clinical considerations for the future.

Keywords: breast cancer, epidemiology, survivors, clinical considerations, forecasting

1. Introduction

In 2015, the World Health Organization reported that cancer ranked within the top four reasons for death, before the age of 70, in 113 of the 172 countries surveyed [1]. The impact of cancer on women's health is incontrovertible. An estimated 2.1 million individuals around the world were diagnosed with breast cancer in 2018, alone [2]. It is the most common malignancy in women, matched only in Sub-Saharan Africa by cervical cancer, due to an elevated prevalence of tumorigenic strains of the human papillomavirus [3].

The breast cancer disease burden is expected to increase, due to a number of socioeconomic risk factors, including: aging and growth of the population, nulliparity, later maternal age at first pregnancy, the use of exogenous hormones (i.e. oral contraceptive pills, hormonal replacement therapy), alcohol intake, and obesity [4].

In addition to this rising incidence rate, outcomes in breast cancer are improving over time. In the United States, mortality has dropped by 40% between 1989 and 2017 [5]. This is thought to be due to a combination of a) mass screening campaigns that allow caregivers to diagnose the disease at earlier stages, thus offering

IntechOpen

better prognoses, and b) the evolution of targeted and increasingly-efficacious therapeutics.

The relative indolence of most non-metastatic breast neoplasms, compared to other malignancies with more acute courses, makes reports of 5-year overall survival less clinically relevant, except in patients who already have limited life expectancy. Additionally, certain breast cancers may be associated with a high rate of late recurrence. For instance, patients with primary tumors that are estrogen receptor (ER)-positive develop distant metastasis in 10–20% of cases, five or more years following initial diagnosis [6]. Therefore, there is great utility in surveying literature, which reports *long-term* survival outcomes in patients with breast cancer. For the purposes of this chapter, we define "long-term survival" as 10-year overall survival (OS).

We start by reporting national data from the United States, and exploring various socio-demographic, clinical, and pathologic characteristics significantly associated with 10-year OS. Next, we perform a literature review of epidemiologic studies from the United States, and around the world, to survey for trends in this growing population. Finally, we explore numerous clinical considerations in addressing the needs of this specific population, with lessons learned from the coronavirus disease 2019 (COVID-19) pandemic, and implications for future clinical care.

2. Prevalence of long-term survivorship in the United States

On an annual basis, the American Cancer Society (ACS) provides national survival data on breast cancer cases diagnosed within the United States. With respect to long-term survival, the society published that current "relative survival rates" for women diagnosed with breast cancer are 85% after 10 years and 80% after 15 years [7]. These rates are age- and race-adjusted; supported by the provided definition of "relative survival" as the "percentage of patients who will survive their cancer for a given period of time after diagnosis...compared to survival among people of the same age and race who have not been diagnosed with cancer" [8]. Despite high heterogeneity within the breast cancer population, the ACS did not stratify long-term survival rates by other socio-demographic, clinical, or pathologic characteristics in this publication. In order to add to ACS findings, we explored the impact of these factors in more granular detail, using OS as reported by the National Cancer Database (NCDB).

The NCDB is a United States-based registry which collects de-identified clinical, pathologic, and outcomes data on approximately 70% of all cancer diagnoses in the country [9]. Data on patients with breast cancer is uploaded into the NCDB from over 1,400 facilities, accredited by the Commission on Cancer and the American College of Surgeons. At the time of this publication, survival surveillance for patients in this repository included data collected through the year 2016. Therefore, in order to ensure adequate time had transpired to capture 10-year OS, we selected a cohort of patients diagnosed between 2004 and 2006. Univariate analysis was conducted to evaluate for independent factors (e.g., age, race, ethnicity, income, insurance status, facility type, co-morbidity index, clinical stage, grade, histology, oncotype, and treatment type) exhibiting significant association with 10-year survival. Subsequently, variables significant at the univariate level were selected for inclusion within one multiple logistic regression model also predicting 10-year survival. A p-value of <0.001 was considered significant, due to the very large sample size that may overpower correlative testing. A total of n = 515,610 patients with breast cancer were analyzed in this model. The results are depicted in **Table 1**, and explained as follows.

Variable	No. (%)	10-year OS				
		%	OR	95% CI		p-value
Age						<.001
<50 (ref)	125,657 (24.4%)	54.1%	1.000	—	—	—
50–70	256,003 (49.7%)	53.0%	.946	.916	.978	.001
>70	133,950 (26.0%)	30.1%	.427	.407	.448	<.001
Race						<.001
White (ref)	440,048 (87.6%)	48.0%	1.000	—	—	—
Black	52,220 (10.4%)	40.7%	.821	.786	.858	<.001
Asian	9872 (2.0%)	51.9%	1.166	1.067	1.275	.001
Ethnicity						
Hispanic (ref)	445,220 (95.6%)	47.7%	1.000	—	—	—
Non-Hispanic	20,481 (4.4%)	44.4%	.936	.878	.998	.042
Income						<.001
<$30,000 (ref)	55,038 (11.0%)	41.8%	1.000	—	—	—
$30,000–$34,999	79,054 (15.8%)	44.9%	1.026	.977	1.078	.296
$35,000–$45,999	133,171 (26.6%)	46.7%	1.065	1.017	1.115	.008
>$46,000	233,078 (46.6%)	50.5%	1.126	1.076	1.178	<.001
Insurance status						<.001
Uninsured (ref)	10,440 (2.1%)	36.8%	1.000	—	—	—
Private insurance	284,063 (56.5%)	55.4%	1.552	1.417	1.701	<.001
Medicare	181,088 (36.0%)	36.5%	1.264	1.150	1.390	<.001
Medicaid/other governmental insurance	26,766 (5.3%)	41.8%	1.211	1.092	1.343	<.001

Variable	No. (%)	10-year OS				
		%	OR	95% CI		p-value
Facility type						<.001
Community cancer program (ref)	46,176 (9.4%)	43.8%	1.000	—	—	—
Comprehensive community cancer program	227,815 (46.5%)	47.7%	1.125	1.077	1.175	<.001
Academic/research program	142,123 (29.0%)	49.0%	1.063	1.015	1.113	.010
Integrated network cancer program	73,703 (15.0%)	44.6%	.819	.776	.865	<.001
Setting						.001
Metro (ref)	427,832 (85.6%)	47.6%	1.000	—	—	—
Urban	63,288 (12.7%)	47.4%	1.076	1.034	1.120	<.001
Rural	8534 (1.7%)	47.4%	1.091	.984	1.209	.099
Charlson/Deyo comorbidity index						.000
0 (ref)	450,329 (87.3%)	49.1%	1.000	—	—	—
1	52,983 (10.3%)	38.3%	.746	.717	.777	<.001
2	9425 (1.8%)	25.1%	.506	.459	.557	<.001
3	2873 (0.6%)	16.4%	.343	.280	.421	<.001
AJCC clinical staging						<.001
0 (ref)	59,736 (25.7%)	54.5%	1.000	—	—	—
1	87,698 (37.7%)	50.0%	.731	.703	.760	<.001
2	51,604 (22.2%)	42.4%	.526	.503	.551	<.001
3	18,871 (8.1%)	29.7%	.281	.264	.299	<.001
4	14,620 (6.3%)	6.1%	.073	.065	.082	<.001
Grade						<.001

DOI: http://dx.doi.org/10.5772/intechopen.95798

Variable	No. (%)	10-year OS				
		%	OR	95% CI		p-value
Well-differentiated (ref)	94,046 (21.2%)	51.6%	1.000	—	—	—
Moderately-differentiated	184,976 (41.7%)	48.5%	.889	.860	.919	<.001
Poorly differentiated	164,490 (37.1%)	44.9%	.782	.752	.812	<.001
Histology						.007
Ductal carcinoma (ref)	367,409 (72.7%)	47.7%	1.000	—	—	—
Lobular carcinoma	79,387 (15.7%)	47.3%	.993	.957	1.031	.720
Other carcinoma	47,959 (9.5%)	49.1%	1.013	.956	1.061	.598
Epithelial-myoepithelial	1861 (0.4%)	42.1%	.898	.703	1.146	.385
Papillary	6005 (1.2%)	30.8%	1.054	.833	1.260	.559
Fibroepithelial	2058 (0.4%)	34.9%	.937	.755	1.162	.552
Mesenchymal	402 (0.1%)	21.4%	.713	0.309	1.645	427
Estrogen receptor status						
Negative (ref)	97,628 (21.9%)	43.9%	1.000	—	—	—
Positive	348,611 (78.1%)	48.6%	.908	.868	.949	<.001
Progesterone receptor status						
Negative (ref)	147,951 (33.6%)	44.0%	1.000	—	—	—
Positive	292,529 (66.4%)	49.3%	1.095	1.057	1.134	<.001
Type of surgery						.000
None (ref)	30,799 (6.0%)	15.8%	1.000	—	—	—
Lumpectomy	294,554 (57.3%)	52.6%	2.300	2.112	2.506	<.001
Mastectomy	188,531 (36.7%)	44.3%	2.320	2.134	2.523	<.001
Radiation						

Variable	No. (%)	10-year OS				
		%	OR	95% CI		p-value
No (ref)	239,355 (47.5%)	40.4%	1.000	—	—	—
Yes	264,681 (52.5%)	53.3%	1.385	1.341	1.430	<.001
Chemotherapy						
No (ref)	309,000 (62.9%)	46.0%	1.000	—	—	—
Yes	182,510 (37.1%)	49.2%	1.375	1.331	1.420	<.001
Hormonal therapy						
No (ref)	245,859 (51.0%)	42.3%	1.000	—	—	—
Yes	236,454 (49.0%)	51.9%	1.207	1.167	1.248	<.001
HER2-targeted therapy						
No (ref)	497,793 (99.6%)	47.2%	1.000	—	—	—
Yes	1862 (0.4%)	43.3%	1.273	1.236	1.311	<.001

Table 1.
Multiple logistic regression model for predictors of long-term overall survival in breast cancer in the United States, using data from the National Cancer Database (NCDB).

2.1 Overall survival by socio-demographic characteristics

Age at diagnosis was significantly associated with likelihood of long-term OS. The age distribution of our cohort was: n = 125,657 (24.4%) <50 years old, n = 256,003 (49.7%) between 50–70 years old, and n = 133,950 (26.0%) older than 70. Long-term OS rates were similar in patients diagnosed before 50 (54.1%) compared to those diagnosed between 50 and 70 years of age (53.0%). This may highlight the relative indolence of breast cancer as a primary malignancy, particularly when diagnosed and treated at early stages. However, a large drop in 10-year OS was seen in those diagnosed after 70 (30.1%), a cohort more likely to experience acute events due to the cumulative effect of chronic comorbidities such as hypertension, diabetes, and dyslipidemia. This is supported by the life expectancy of individuals in the United States which, in 2016, was estimated to be 78.9 years [10]. The distribution of survival, by age, may differ in other parts of the world, particularly in low- and middle-income countries, or those without mass screening programs.

Racial disparities continue to be a significant major healthcare challenge. In the 1980s, a marked divergence in death rates between White and Black women with breast cancer was first noted [11]. The implementation of mass screening programs disproportionately benefited areas wherein residents had access to favorably-resourced and accredited healthcare institutions [12, 13]; these communities were predominantly White. Additionally, hormonal therapy (e.g. tamoxifen), newly introduced to systemic treatment regimens for treatment of ER+ tumors, was not appropriate for many Black women, who are more likely to present with triple negative breast cancer (TNBC) – a type of breast cancer without ER, PR, or HER2 expression, which is unresponsive to tamoxifen regimens [14]. This is elaborated upon in Section 2.2.

Race-based survival disparity peaked in 2011, with mortality rates reported to be approximately 45% higher in Black versus White patients with breast cancer [5]. Despite improvements over the last decade, race continues to be an important predictor of 10-year OS ($p < 0.001$), as depicted in **Figure 1**. In our analysis, using data extrapolated from the NCDB, patients of Asian descent exhibited the highest long-term overall survival rate (51.9%), followed by White (48.0%) and then Black (40.7%) patients. Beyond access to healthcare, these race-based disparities are thought to be due to the complex interplay between multiple lifestyle factors (such as alcohol consumption and smoking), extent of comorbidity (including obesity, which is associated with worse outcomes in breast cancer due to increased estrogens and inflammatory mediators [15]), and genetics. Interestingly, from our analysis, ethnicity (defined in the NCDB as Hispanic vs. Non-Hispanic) was not determined to be a significant predictor of 10-year OS, even when adjusting for

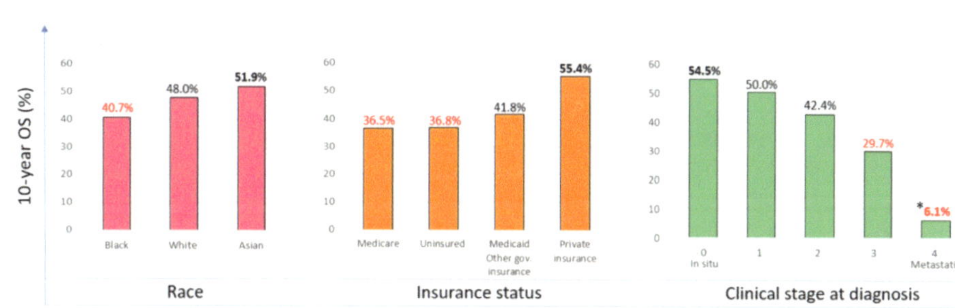

Figure 1.
Pictorial of key predictors of 10-year OS in the United States, through analysis of the National Cancer Database (NCDB).

relevant confounders such as age, race, comorbidity (Charlson/Deyo index), and AJCC clinical stage at diagnosis.

Measures of socioeconomic status – including annual income, insurance status, and treatment facility type – were also significantly associated with 10-year OS in this cohort ($p < 0.001$). Patients who were uninsured exhibited the lowest 10-year OS rates (36.8%), in contrast to patients who had private insurance (56.5%), as depicted in **Figure 1**. A study by Ko, et al., indicates that roughly half of all racial/ethnic disparity, associated with the risk of locally-advanced disease, can be attributed to insurance status as "uninsured" or "underinsured" [16]. Patients without healthcare coverage are less likely to effectively manage chronic comorbidities, including hypertension [17] and diabetes [18], which is likely a contributing factor of higher mortality observed in this subgroup. While setting (urban vs. rural) was not a significant predictor of long-term survival, facility type was ($p < 0.001$), with patients treated at academic cancer programs exhibiting the highest 10-year OS rate (49.0%), followed by those treated at comprehensive community cancer programs (47.7%) and those treated at community cancer programs (43.8%). This may be due to differences in time-to-diagnosis and time-to-treatment, determined by institution size, and care practices that may differ based on the accreditation of different cancer programs, as available to different communities [19].

2.2 Overall survival by clinical characteristics

As expected, the most important predictor of survival in breast cancer in our analysis was 'stage' at diagnosis, as depicted in **Figure 1**. Breast cancer stage represents the extent of spread of cancer in the body, expressed on a spectrum ranging from 0 (the earliest form, wherein cancer cells are restricted to the milk ducts of the breast, but have not invaded other breast tissue) to IV (the latest form, where the cancer has spread to another organ in the body, referred to as "metastatic"). Staging may be *clinical* (based on physical exam and imaging such as mammogram, ultrasound, or magnetic resonance imaging) or *pathologic* (based on evaluation of breast tissue and lymph nodes removed during surgery). We found that the widest disparity in long-term OS was associated with clinical stage of diagnosis (54.5% with stage 0, versus just 6.1% with stage IV disease, $p < 0.001$). As the majority of patients in the United States are diagnosed at early stages of disease (i.e. 0-II), this supports the positive, clinical impact of public health campaigns that target awareness of prevalence, risk factors, signs and symptoms of breast cancer.

Diagnosis of breast cancer is typically confirmed with a biopsy, during which a tumor tissue sample is sent for evaluation by specialists in pathology. Through microscopy, and the use of staining techniques, numerous pathophysiological characteristics of the neoplasm can be determined. Important among them, is the 'breast cancer subtype', referring to the molecular profile of the tumor, based on the expression of three receptors on the surface of breast cancer cells: 1) the estrogen receptor (ER), 2) progesterone receptor (PR), and the 3) human epidermal factor growth factor 2 (HER2) receptor. The combination of these receptors forms the basis for clinical decision-making regarding targeted therapy in breast cancer. For instance, if the primary tumor is ER+/PR+, 'endocrine' or 'hormonal' therapy can be administered (e.g. selective estrogen receptor modulators, or SERMs, like tamoxifen, that directly modulate these hormonal receptors, or aromatase inhibitors, which decrease the natural conversion of androgens to estrogens in the body); if the tumor exhibits HER2+ status, the monoclonal antibody trastuzumab is given to block this receptor subtype.

The NCDB did not routinely document HER2 receptor status in cases diagnosed before 2009, thus the impact of this receptor expression on 10-year OS could not be evaluated in this multivariate model. However, the analysis did include ER status and PR status, demonstrating that positivity of either receptor significantly predicted long-term survival. This finding underscores progress made in the improvement of patient outcomes as treatment modalities become more targeted (prior to endocrine therapy, non-targeted chemotherapy was the gold standard for treatment of even hormone receptor positive breast cancer). This is also strongly reflected in one of our previous analyses, indicating that patients with tumors which were negative for all three receptors (TNBC), exhibited the lowest rate of 5-year OS (71%), followed by the ER-, PR-, HER2+ subtype (77%), the ER/PR+, HER2+ subtype (83%), and a highest 5-year OS rate seen in the ER/PR+, HER2- subtype (84%) [20].

Interestingly, HER2 overexpression, occurring in around 20% of breast cancers, is associated with worse natural prognosis due to increased growth and marked metastatic potential of these tumors [21]. However, we have shown that survival outcomes in ER/PR-, HER2+ breast cancer, in the United States, have surpassed TNBC due to the advent of HER2-targeted regimens. Therefore, HER2+ status may be predictive of treatment efficacy in breast cancer. This may not be the case globally, particularly in low- and middle-income countries which may exhibit limitation in drug funding. In 2012, the Union for International Cancer Control and the Dana-Farber Cancer Institute filed an application with the World Health Organization to add trastuzumab (a HER2-targeted therapy) to the essential medications list [22], an advisory list of the minimum medicine needs for basic healthcare systems. This was not approved until May 2015 [23]. Current literature still reports trans-national disparities in the availability of HER2-targeted therapeutics, and advocates for the distribution of more affordable trastuzumab biosimilars in order to address this ongoing need [24, 25].

Pathologists will also assign a 'grade' to the tumor under evaluation using a method of classification known as the Nottingham modification of the Scarff-Bloom-Richardson system [26]. Grading in breast cancer designates how "abnormal" neoplastic cells appear, and is based on the extent of glandular/tubular differentiation, nuclear pleomorphism, and mitotic count [27]. Grade 1 tumors are "well differentiated", meaning their growth is slower and appears most similarly to normal breast tissue. Grade 3 tumors, on the other hand, are "poorly differentiated", appearing "dysplastic" (very different from normal cells) and have a higher growth potential. Grade 2, tumors have "moderate" differentiation, and fall between Grade 1 and Grade 3 in prognostic implication. While not predictive of the same breadth of overall survivorship as tumor staging, we found in our NCDB analysis that tumor grade was still a statistically significant predictor of 10-year OS: patients with Grade 1 tumors exhibited a 10-year OS rate of 51.6% (unadjusted for stage at diagnosis) versus those with Grade 2 tumors (48.5%) and those with Grade 3 tumors (44.9%). Finally, we also showed that while 'histological subtype' (referring to the tissue type a neoplasm originated from) was not a statistically-significant predictor of long-term overall survival ($p > 0.001$), the highest 10-year OS rates were seen in the most common subtypes: ductal carcinoma (47.7%, not adjusted for stage at diagnosis) and lobular carcinoma (47.3%). Patients with some rare histologies exhibited lower rates of 10-year OS, including epithelial-myoepithelial (42.1%), fibroepithelial (34.9%), papillary (30.8%), and mesenchymal (21.4%) breast cancers. The scarcity of these subtypes has limited the ability to study these unique histologies in a high-throughput manner. However, recent studies suggest that tumor histology should be considered when determining the optimal treatment approach for each patient [28–30].

3. Prevalence of long-term survivorship globally

Survival rates for breast cancer vary considerably in different parts of the world. The 5-year OS rate – which is more commonly reported and can thus be compared when controlling for confounders such as race, stage at diagnosis, age at diagnosis, etc. – varies from over 80% in developed countries, to less than 60% in low- and middle-income countries [31]. However, less is known about 10-year OS in low- and middle-income countries. We conducted a systematic search using MEDLINE, via PubMed and Google Scholar, from inception until December 2020. We included observational cohort studies also reporting OS rates if published in the English language. The search strategy involved a combination of free text searches, as well as medical subject headings (MeSH), as follows: ("Breast Neoplasms" [MeSH], OR "breast cancer" OR "breast tumor") AND ("Survival" [MeSH] OR "Survival Rate" [MeSH] OR "Life Tables" [MeSH] OR "Kaplan–Meier Estimate" [MeSH] OR "Hazard Ratio" OR "Cox regression") AND ("Cohort Studies" [MeSH] OR "Retrospective Studies" [MeSH] or "Prospective Studies" [MeSH] OR "follow-up" or "longitude").

We found n = 37 studies reporting 10-year OS rates, as presented in **Table 2**. The majority were from high income countries (n = 27, 73%), while n = 10 (27%) reported data from low- and middle-income countries. It was found that high income countries have been reporting long-term OS data over a longer period of time (1978–2020), while data from low- and middle-income countries have been published more recently (2008–2020). Additionally, cohorts used in studies from high income countries were larger (mean sample size: n = 1,573) than those from low- and middle-income countries (mean sample size: n = 268). In comparing data published since the year 2000, the mean 10-year OS rate from high-income country studies was 72%, versus the mean 10-year OS rate from low- and middle-income countries studies, which was 64%. However, these comparisons do not control for the impact of patients age at diagnosis (most studies did not report a

First author	Year of publication	Country	Sample size	Mean age y +/– SD	10-year survival
Low- and middle-income countries					
Mai TTX et al.	2019	Korea	206	47 +/– 9	0.88
Dolatkhah R et al	2019	Iran	4989	50.4 +/– 13	0.65
Bender MPF et al	2015	Brazil	264	63 +/– 13	0.41
Ziaei JE et al	2013	Iran	271	48	0.76
Li BJ et al	2012	China	84	57 +/– 11	0.63
Gokce T et al	2011	Turkey	1746	51	0.79
Xia LP et al	2010	China	70	NR	0.73
Heydari ST et al	2009	Iran	877	47 +/– 12	0.46
Rajaeefard AR et al	2009	Iran	310	NR	0.53
Yaghmaei et al	2008	Iran	50	52 +/– 14	0.47
High-income countries					
Wu SC et al	2020	Taiwan	2,002	NR	0.78
Ameijide A et al	2019	Spain	10,195	NR	0.41

First author	Year of publication	Country	Sample size	Mean age y +/− SD	10-year survival
Ignatov A et al	2018	Germany	12,053	NR	0.82
Yoshimura A et al	2018	Japan	63,348	NR	0.79
Park EH et al	2017	Korea	109,988	NR	0.85
Plichta JK et al	2016	USA	584	NR	0.86
Campbell ID et al	2015	New Zealand	101,824	NR	0.84
Fong Y et al	2014	England	1,712	NR	0.77
Hamadeh RR et al	2014	Bahrain	1,005	51	0.49
Hauth EA et al	2012	Germany	222	NR	0.96
Marchal F et al	2009	France	116	66 +/− 12	0.52
Thalib L ct al	2009	Sweden	300,011	NR	0.64
Ueno M et al	2007	Japan	559	NR	0.75
Jayasinghe UW et al	2005	Australia	393	54	0.69
Tejler G et al	2004	Sweden	7,892	NR	0.54
Minelli L et al	2004	Italy	2,460	NR	0.47
Jensen AR et al	2003	Denmark	1,573	56	0.66
Twelves CJ et al	2001	Scotland	1,617	NR	0.52
Barchielli A et al	1999	Italy	1,182	NR	0.53
Fakhro AE et al	1999	Bahrain	93	50	0.36
Wallgren A et al	1997	Sweden	75	NR	0.54
Sariego J et al	1995	USA	81	NR	0.49
Sant M et al	1991	Italy	1,991	NR	0.5
Toikkanen S et al	1990	Finland	461	NR	0.37
Isard HJ et al.	1988	USA	70	57	0.7
Adami HO et al	1985	Sweden	12,319	NR	0.38
Heller KS et al	1978	USA	304	65	0.62

Table 2.
Review of global cohort data reporting long-term overall survival rates of breast cancer.

mean age), disease stage at diagnosis (though all cohorts reported individuals from all four stages of breast cancer), race, or the presence of comorbidities in these cohorts. Therefore, more information will be needed to calculate pooled estimates of global survival, by region or country. This review of studies reveals a stark disparity in the availability of long-term outcomes data from different regions around the world.

4. Forecasting stage of diagnosis in the United States to 2030

As mentioned, the strongest predictor of 10-year survival outcomes, in breast cancer, is stage at diagnosis. As diagnostic capabilities continue to facilitate earlier identification of disease, it is important to understand how stage migration is predicted to change in the future – an important metric for allocation of resources and services needed for this growing group of survivors.

In order to understand future stage migration patterns, in a cohort of long-term survivors of breast cancer, there is utility in forecasting the predicted proportion of cases that are expected to be early stage (0, I or II) versus late stage (III or IV) based on historical trends. To do this, we extracted annual incidence data from the NCDB from 2004–2016, stratifying by cases that were diagnosed at early stage versus those at late stages. This data was analyzed via time-series forecasting, specifically autoregressive integrated moving averages (ARIMA) modeling, which considers annual variation and accounts for temporal correlation in analysis of historical data [32]. The performance of ARIMA models has been found to be comparable to other time series models in its capacity to forecast healthcare data, such as the Bayesian shared two-component model [33].

Multiple ARIMA models were generated using the Statistical Package for the Social Sciences (SPSS) Version 27.0 software (IBM Corp, Armonk, NY) using different combinations of the autoregressive parameters for 'p', the order of the autoregressive model, 'd', the degree of differencing and 'q', the order of the moving average (p, d, q). The most predictive model was selected using the lowest Bayesian Information Criteria, and mean absolute percentage error, and this was the (0, 1, 0) ARIMA model. **Figure 2** depicts 1) the historical incidence of breast cancer in the United States (black curve), stratified by stage at diagnosis (blue for early-stage and red for late-stage) for the years 2004–2016, and 2) forecasted incidence of total, early stage and late stage cases to the year 2030. The annual proportion of new cases diagnosed at late-stage is highlighted on as an emboldened numerical figure in red. Tabulated numerical data of these forecasts can be found in **Table 3**.

We found that, based on historical trends, the proportion of cases diagnosed at advanced stages of disease is projected to fall to 10.7%, compared to the historical proportion, in 2004, of 19.8%. Based on this projected stage migration, we can expect the number of long-term survivors in the United States to continue to grow. In Section 5, we discuss the impact of the COVID-19 pandemic on mass screening, and implications for staging and care of patients diagnosed during 2020.

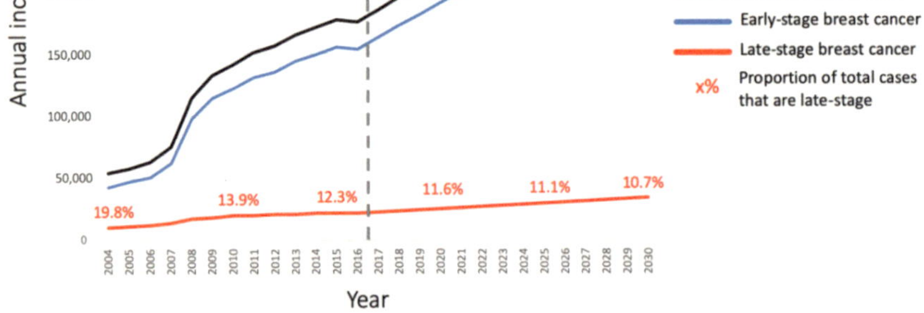

Figure 2.
ARIMA forecasts of breast cancer incidence in the United States to the year 2030, stratified by stage at diagnosis, using the NCDB.

	Year	Total Incidence	Incidence Diagnosed at Early Stages (0–2)	Incidence Diagnosed at Late Stages [3–4]	% of Cases Diagnosed at Advanced Stages
Historical data from the NCDB	2004	53,551	42,970	10,581	19.76%
	2005	57,902	46,792	11,110	19.19%
	2006	62,412	50,503	11,909	19.08%
	2007	75,251	61,786	13,465	17.89%
	2008	114,666	97,699	16,967	14.80%
	2009	132,520	114,357	18,163	13.71%
	2010	141,328	121,716	19,612	13.88%
	2011	151,081	130,967	20,114	13.31%
	2012	156,102	135,506	20,596	13.19%
	2013	164,902	143,840	21,062	12.77%
	2014	171,275	149,422	21,353	12.76%
	2015	177,569	155,709	21,860	12.31%
	2016	175,293	153,924	21,369	12.19%

	Year	Total Incidence	Incidence Diagnosed at Early Stages (0–2)	Incidence Diagnosed at Late Stages [3–4]	% of Cases Diagnosed at Advanced Stages
Forecasted data using (0,1,0) ARIMA modeling	2017	185,438	163,170	22,268	12.01%
	2018	195,583	172,416	23,167	11.85%
	2019	205,728	181,662	24,066	11.70%
	2020	215,873	190,908	24,965	11.56%
	2021	226,018	200,154	25,864	11.44%
	2022	236,164	209,401	26,763	11.33%
	2023	246,309	218,647	27,662	11.23%
	2024	256,454	227,893	28,561	11.14%
	2025	266,599	237,139	29,460	11.05%
	2026	276,744	246,385	30,359	10.97%
	2027	286,889	255,631	31,258	10.90%
	2028	297,035	264,878	32,157	10.83%
	2029	307,180	274,124	33,056	10.76%
	2030	317,325	283,370	33,955	10.70%

Table 3.
Historical incidence and forecasted incidence to 2030 of breast cancer in the United States, using data from the National Cancer Database (NCDB).

5. Impact of the COVID-19 pandemic

5.1 COVID-19: Epidemiology & healthcare impacts

The COVID-19 pandemic is now a defining feature of the year 2020. This novel coronavirus was identified in 2019, as the etiology of a pneumonia diagnosis in Wuhan, in the Hubei province in China [34]. Genomic sequencing and phylogenetic analysis indicated that the coronavirus that causes COVID-19 is of the same subgenus as the severe acute respiratory syndrome (SARS) virus [35, 36]. This led to the determination that COVID-19 is due to severe acute respiratory syndrome coronarivurs-2. Following its discovery, the outbreak of this disease spread rapidly: on January 10, 2020, the genomic sequence of SARS-CoV-2 was released and shared globally by China [37]; by February of 2020, COVID-19 had quickly spread through the Hubei province [38]; and On March 11,2020, the World Health Organization, had declared the COVID-19 outbreak a global emergency and pandemic [38].

In an attempt to flatten the epidemiologic growth curve of new COVID-19 diagnoses, public health departments implemented targeted social measures to decrease transmission rates. This included emphasis on social distancing, stay-at-home mandates, a requirement of face masks worn in public, and hand hygiene [39]. Additionally, in order to reduce mortality and relieve the case-load pressure on clinical care providers, many healthcare systems were forced to change clinical practice. While there has been much investigation into the pathology and biologic effects of COVID-19, the overall impact of COVID-19 on management of chronic health outcomes – including breast cancer management and overall survival – is still evolving.

Due to the COVID-19 pandemic, the mechanism for healthcare delivery has changed substantially. One of the changes seen in the United States, was the broad adoption of telemedicine and the upheaval of the in-person visit. Prior to the year 2020, the use of telemedicine was unsubstantial [40]. However, telemedicine visits increased from 1.1% during the second quarter (Q2) of 2019, to 35.3% in Q2 of 2020 [41]. Correspondingly, as the rise in the rate of remote visits increased, the number of in-person visits decreased – the number of office-based health care visits in Q2 of 2020, decreased by 50.2% compared with the previous year [41]. While helping to slow the dissemination of COVID-19, this decrease of in-person visits has made the full-spectrum of care for patients with breast cancer challenging, because physical exams and in-person evaluations have also declined. As a result, co-morbidity management may have also suffered: during Q2 of 2020, blood pressure assessments decreased by 50.1%, while cholesterol assessments decreased by 35.3% [41].

The overall effect of COVID-19 on delays in cancer diagnosis, disruptions in treatment, and modifications to therapeutic regimens is still being evaluated. One report, including 609 patients with breast cancer, identified treatment delays for 44% of the study population, aged 45 years and younger [42]. Another study suggests a higher death rate in cancer patients in receipt of recent therapy, however the proportion of patients reported on active therapy, in this study, was marginal and thus conclusive correlation cannot be determined [43–45]. Literature has shown that patients with cancer, when compared to those without cancer, are at increased susceptibility to infection, secondary to systemic immunosuppression from their cancer or anticancer therapy [46–49]. Initial reports suggested patients with cancer experienced more frequent COVID-19 complications [43, 50, 51]. As a result, physicians and patients must strategically balance the risks of cancer advancement, cancer relapse, etc. with the risks of hospitalization or death secondary to a COVID-19-related complication. Through diagnoses to management, special concern for patients with cancer is warranted due to the pandemic.

Patients with breast cancer might be at an increased risk for treatment-related complications and other health issues during the COVID-19 pandemic. The CDC reports that having cancer increases your risk of severe illness from COVID-19 [52]. Several studies have been conducted with respect to the effects of COVID-19 on patients with cancer. One multicenter study was conducted to evaluate the clinical characteristics of COVID-19-infected patients who died within 28 days of hospitalization in the intensive care unit [53]. This study reported 784 deaths after 28 days, 60 of these deaths (7.7%) were among those with active cancer; their multivariable model revealed that active cancer was associated with increased COVID-19-driven mortality (odds ratio (OR), 2.15; 95% CI, 1.35–3.43) [53]. An additional multi-institutional study was performed to evaluate the impact of COVID-19 on patients with active or prior malignancies [54]. The primary end point of this analysis was all-cause mortality, within 30 days of a COVID-19 diagnosis. Within this population, 22% had hematologic malignancies, and the remainder were previously diagnosed with solid tumors [54]. This study did *not* find an association between increased COVID-19-related mortality and cancer type, anticancer therapy, or recent surgery. There were several factors associated with increased 30-day mortality: male sex (OR, 1.63 [95% CI, 1.07–2.48]), older age (per 10 years) (partially adjusted OR, 1.84 [95% CI, 1.53–2.21]), increased comorbidities (≥2) (OR, 4.50 [95% CI, 1.33–15.28]), a previous smoking status (OR, 1.60 [95% CI, 1.03–2.47]), Eastern Cooperative Oncology Group performance status 2 (OR, 3.89 [95% CI, 2.11–7.18]) or more (OR, 5.66 [95% CI, 2.79–11.47]), and progressive cancer (defined as no longer responding to treatment) (OR, 5.20 [95% CI, 2.77–9.77]) [54].

5.2 Relationship between COVID-19 and breast cancer

The increased risk of severe illness, secondary to COVID-19, in patients with breast cancer [52] might be multifaceted. Both cancer, and cancer treatment, can cause a significant physiologic strain on protective mechanisms of the human body. The immune system is intrinsically linked to breast cancer pathogenesis via inflammatory pathways, immune surveillance, and adaptive immunity [55]. Chronic inflammatory activity has been discovered in all breast cancers, regardless of breast cancer subtype [56]. This chronic inflammation can lead to damaged breast cells, which may support continued tumor progression, with some breast cancer models revealing CD4+ T lymphocytes indirectly promoting invasion and metastasis [57].

An additional reason for a potentially increased risk of serious complications, including death, secondary to COVID-19, in breast cancer patients, is impaired immunity due to chemotherapy. Treatment, with chemotherapy or radiation therapy, can lead to chronic pain, immune suppression, treatment-related toxicities, failure to thrive, and decreased physical and cognitive abilities [58]. Chemotherapy has been shown to induce neutropenia and lymphopenia in patients [59]. Women with breast cancer, who were treated with adjuvant therapy that consisted of chlorambucil, methotrexate, and 5-fluorouracil had decreased peripheral blood lymphocytes [60]. Similarly, other studies report decreased CD4+ cell counts along with concurrent pneumocystis pneumonia in patients with breast cancer who had received multi-agent chemotherapy and radiation therapy [61].

The relationship between the uses of immune check point inhibitors (ICIs) in breast cancer patients is another new area of interest during the COVID-19 pandemic. Several ICIs have been developed targeting breast cancer; some of the most clinically-advanced are those that target programmed cell death-1 (PD-1) and programmed cell death ligand-1 (PD-L1) [62]. Anti-PD-1/PD-L1 agents are an emerging treatment modality with encouraging results for aggressive breast tumors, like triple negative breast cancers [63]. These ICI therapies, however, are associated with several significant side effects -- one of which includes inflammatory syndromes like pneumonitis, which targets the lungs [64, 65]. These treatments have also been associated with increased inflammation and tissue damage [66, 67]. Currently, reports evaluating the relationship between anti-PD-1/PD-L1 agents and COVID-19 are ongoing. But, some preclinical studies reveal that viral clearance is accelerated by PD-1/PDL-1 pathways and, thus blocked by immune check point inhibitors [68]. Other reports have associated COVD-19 with increased T-cell exhaustion when there is increased expression of PD-1 and PDL-1 [69].

As the effect of COVID-19 on breast cancer patients in receipt of ICIs is still being evaluated, members of the medical community defer to historical trends between ICIs and other viruses for clinical decision making. For instance, the checkpoint inhibitor, pembrolizumab has demonstrated efficacy in a subset of patients with progressive multifocal leukoencephalopathy caused by JC virus infection [70]. Additionally, some studies have noted that ICIs exacerbate viral lung infections, with increased toxicities observed in the winter months when the majority of the population are diagnosed with colds and the flu [71, 72].

Although there are increased risks and side effects associated with the use of chemotherapy and ICIs during the COVID-19 pandemic, the benefits of these treatment modalities could outweigh the risks. The OS of breast cancer patients has improved significantly over the last three decades, due in part to improvements in systemic chemotherapy, endocrine therapy, targeted therapy, and recently the application of ICIs [73, 74]. Therefore, while breast cancer therapies may be associated with negative side effects, recovery is possible with appropriate management, dependent upon tumor burden and the overall health status of the patient [75–77]. In order to maximize the clinical efficacy of these treatment modalities, while limiting COVID-19-related health risks, additional research is needed to guide practice.

6. Clinical considerations of a growing cohort of long-term survivors

While outcomes following treatment of invasive breast cancer have become increasingly favorable, survivors remain at-risk for recurrence of disease, either loco-regionally or at a distant site. In one large cohort of 9,514 women diagnosed with breast cancer under the age of 75, 10.4% developed distant metastasis, most commonly at a bony site [78]. Patients were more likely to experience recurrence in the period 5–10 years after diagnosis, if they presented with primary tumors that were ER-positive, lymph-node positive, or larger than 20 mm in size [78]. Women with ER-negative tumors, however, have a lower risk during this period. The development of multigene sequencing panels predicting outcomes in ER-positive tumors can guide clinicians to ensure at-risk patients receive the appropriate adjuvant therapy.

Survivors of breast cancer should undergo regular follow-up for surveillance and management of treatment-related effects, as well as breast-specific and other indicated imaging to evaluate for malignant recurrence, or new disease. This management necessarily includes a wide range of disciplines in medicine. Breast surgery or radiation therapy can result in chronic pain, fibrosis, fat necrosis, or recurrent skin infections in the chest wall [79, 80]. Patients are also at long-term-risk for cardiovascular dysfunction, including congestive heart failure [81], ovarian failure [82], and even the development of secondary cancers [83]. For this reason, the care of long-term survivors of breast cancer should be based on collaboration between multiple subspecialties. Patients should also continue to receive age-appropriate screening as indicated for the general population with respect to conditions other than breast cancer.

Cancer diagnoses are also associated with increased patient distress and anxiety [84]. Therefore, clinicians are strongly encouraged to consider psychosocial support for long-term breast cancer survivors, as an important complement to clinical monitoring. Providing integrated care that is directed to the overall wellness of the patient, maximizes the potential to increase patient satisfaction, increase patient medical compliance, and preserve quality of life [85–87]. Interestingly, it has also been found that ethnic minority groups, who typically report poorer quality of life and worse distress after diagnosis, may derive more acute benefit from integrated modalities like art therapy [88]. It is also of importance to note that effective psychosocial support programs have been shown to be significantly associated with favorable clinical outcomes [84, 89–92].

7. Conclusions

The advancement of screening modalities and novel therapies has led to more favorable prognoses in patients with breast cancer. As a result, long-term breast cancer survivors are a large and continually-growing group, globally. This group is also projected to increase, substantially, within coming years. While these trends are favorable and clinically promising, patients with breast cancer should undergo regular follow-up for surveillance and management of treatment-related effects, as well as potential disease recurrence. In the time of the COVID-19 pandemic, it is also important to note a potential combinatorial effect of possible complications secondary to cancer treatment received, and possible impact on screening and treatment delays imposed by the novel coronavirus, on both communities and health care delivery systems.

Conflict of interest

The authors declare no conflict of interest.

Abbreviations

ACS	American Cancer Society
ARIMA	Autroregressive integrated moving average
COVID-19	Coronavirus disease 2019
ER	Estrogen receptor
HER2	Human epidermal growth factor 2
ICI	Immune checkpoint inhibitor
NCDB	National Cancer Database
OS	Overall survival
PR	Progesterone receptor
PD-1	Programmed cell death-1
PD-L1	Programmed cell death ligand
SARS	Severe acute respiratory disorder
TNBC	Triple negative breast cancer

Author details

Nadeem Bilani, Elizabeth Blessing Elimimian, Leah Elson, Hong Liang and Zeina Nahleh*
Cleveland Clinic Florida, Weston, Florida, USA

*Address all correspondence to: nahlehz@ccf.org

References

[1] World Health Organization. Global Health Estimates: Life expectancy and leading causes of death and disability. https://www.who.int/data/gho/data/themes/mortality-and-global-health-estimates. Accessed on December 10, 2020.

[2] Bray F, Ferlay J, Soerjomataram I, Siegel RL, Torre LA, Jemal A. Global cancer statistics 2018: GLOBOCAN estimates of incidence and mortality worldwide for 36 cancers in 185 countries. CA Cancer J Clin. 2018;68(6):394-424.

[3] Jedy-Agba E, Joko WY, Liu B, Buziba NG, Borok M, Korir A, et al. Trends in cervical cancer incidence in sub-Saharan Africa. Br J Cancer. 2020;123(1):148-54.

[4] Lundqvist A, Andersson E, Ahlberg I, Nilbert M, Gerdtham U. Socioeconomic inequalities in breast cancer incidence and mortality in Europe-a systematic review and meta-analysis. European journal of public health. 2016;26(5):804-13.

[5] DeSantis CE, Ma J, Gaudet MM, Newman LA, Miller KD, Sauer AG, et al. Breast cancer statistics, 2019. CA: A Cancer Journal for Clinicians. 2019.

[6] Zhang XHF, Giuliano M, Trivedi MV, Schiff R, Osborne CK. Metastasis dormancy in estrogen receptor-positive breast cancer. Clinical cancer research : an official journal of the American Association for Cancer Research. 2013;19(23):6389-97.

[7] American Cancer Society. Breast Cancer Facts & Figures 2019-2020. https://www.cancer.org/content/dam/cancer-org/research/cancer-facts-and-statistics/breast-cancer-facts-and-figures/breast-cancer-facts-and-figures-2019-2020.pdf. Accessed on December 10, 2020.

[8] Zavala VA, Bracci PM, Carethers JM, Carvajal-Carmona L, Coggins NB, Cruz-Correa MR, et al. Cancer health disparities in racial/ethnic minorities in the United States. British journal of cancer. 2020.

[9] Bilimoria KY, Stewart AK, Winchester DP, Ko CY. The National Cancer Data Base: a powerful initiative to improve cancer care in the United States. Annals of surgical oncology. 2008;15(3):683-90.

[10] Woolf SH, Schoomaker H. Life Expectancy and Mortality Rates in the United States, 1959-2017. Jama. 2019;322(20):1996-2016.

[11] Richardson LC, Henley SJ, Miller JW, Massetti G, Thomas CC. Patterns and Trends in Age-Specific Black-White Differences in Breast Cancer Incidence and Mortality - United States, 1999-2014. MMWR Morb Mortal Wkly Rep. 2016;65(40):1093-8.

[12] Warnecke RB, Campbell RT, Vijayasiri G, Barrett RE, Rauscher GH. Multilevel Examination of Health Disparity: The Role of Policy Implementation in Neighborhood Context, in Patient Resources, and in Healthcare Facilities on Later Stage of Breast Cancer Diagnosis. Cancer Epidemiol Biomarkers Prev. 2019;28(1):59-66.

[13] Molina Y, Silva A, Rauscher GH. Racial/Ethnic Disparities in Time to a Breast Cancer Diagnosis: The Mediating Effects of Health Care Facility Factors. Med Care. 2015;53(10):872-8.

[14] Stead LA, Lash TL, Sobieraj JE, Chi DD, Westrup JL, Charlot M, et al. Triple-negative breast cancers are increased in black women regardless of age or body mass index. Breast Cancer Res. 2009;11(2):R18.

[15] Picon-Ruiz M, Morata-Tarifa C, Valle-Goffin JJ, Friedman ER, Slingerland JM. Obesity and adverse breast cancer risk and outcome: Mechanistic insights and strategies for intervention. CA: a cancer journal for clinicians. 2017;67(5):378-97.

[16] Ko NY, Hong S, Winn RA, Calip GS. Association of Insurance Status and Racial Disparities With the Detection of Early-Stage Breast Cancer. JAMA Oncology. 2020;6(3):385-92.

[17] Egan BM, Li J, Small J, Nietert PJ, Sinopoli A. The growing gap in hypertension control between insured and uninsured adults: National Health and Nutrition Examination Survey 1988 to 2010. Hypertension. 2014;64(5):997-1004.

[18] Zhang X, Bullard KM, Gregg EW, Beckles GL, Williams DE, Barker LE, et al. Access to health care and control of ABCs of diabetes. Diabetes Care. 2012;35(7):1566-71.

[19] Bleicher RJ. Timing and Delays in Breast Cancer Evaluation and Treatment. Annals of surgical oncology. 2018;25(10):2829-38.

[20] Bilani N, Zabor EC, Elson L, Elimimian EB, Nahleh Z. Breast Cancer in the United States: A Cross-Sectional Overview. J Cancer Epidemiol. 2020;2020:6387378-.

[21] Arteaga CL, Sliwkowski MX, Osborne CK, Perez EA, Puglisi F, Gianni L. Treatment of HER2-positive breast cancer: current status and future perspectives. Nat Rev Clin Oncol. 2011;9(1):16-32.

[22] Ruff P, Al-Sukhun S, Blanchard C, Shulman LN. Access to Cancer Therapeutics in Low- and Middle-Income Countries. Am Soc Clin Oncol Educ Book. 2016;35:58-65.

[23] Gray AL, Wirtz VJ, t Hoen EF, Reich MR, Hogerzeil HV. Essential medicines are still essential. Lancet. 2015;386(10004):1601-3.

[24] Blackwell K, Gligorov J, Jacobs I, Twelves C. The Global Need for a Trastuzumab Biosimilar for Patients With HER2-Positive Breast Cancer. Clinical breast cancer. 2018;18(2):95-113.

[25] Cortes J, Perez-García JM, Llombart-Cussac A, Curigliano G, El Saghir NS, Cardoso F, et al. Enhancing global access to cancer medicines. CA Cancer J Clin. 2020;70(2):105-24.

[26] Elston CW, Ellis IO. Pathological prognostic factors in breast cancer. I. The value of histological grade in breast cancer: experience from a large study with long-term follow-up. Histopathology. 1991;19(5):403-10.

[27] Rabe K, Snir OL, Bossuyt V, Harigopal M, Celli R, Reisenbichler ES. Interobserver variability in breast carcinoma grading results in prognostic stage differences. Hum Pathol. 2019;94:51-7.

[28] Lobbezoo D, Truin W, Voogd A, Roumen R, Vreugdenhil G, Dercksen MW, et al. The role of histological subtype in hormone receptor positive metastatic breast cancer: similar survival but different therapeutic approaches. Oncotarget. 2016;7(20):29412-9.

[29] Akiyama F, Horii R. Therapeutic strategies for breast cancer based on histological type. Breast Cancer. 2009;16(3):168-72.

[30] Singh K, He X, Kalife ET, Ehdaivand S, Wang Y, Sung CJ. Relationship of histologic grade and histologic subtype with oncotype Dx recurrence score; retrospective review of 863 breast cancer oncotype

Dx results. Breast Cancer Res Treat. 2018;168(1):29-34.

[31] Coleman MP, Quaresma M, Berrino F, Lutz JM, De Angelis R, Capocaccia R, et al. Cancer survival in five continents: a worldwide population-based study (CONCORD). Lancet Oncol. 2008;9(8):730-56.

[32] Earnest A, Evans SM, Sampurno F, Millar J. Forecasting annual incidence and mortality rate for prostate cancer in Australia until 2022 using autoregressive integrated moving average (ARIMA) models. BMJ Open. 2019;9(8):e031331-e.

[33] Earnest A, Tan SB, Wilder-Smith A, Machin D. Comparing statistical models to predict dengue fever notifications. Comput Math Methods Med. 2012;2012:758674.

[34] Zheng J. SARS-CoV-2: an emerging coronavirus that causes a global threat. International journal of biological sciences. 2020;16(10):1678.

[35] Lu R, Zhao X, Li J, Niu P, Yang B, Wu H, et al. Genomic characterisation and epidemiology of 2019 novel coronavirus: implications for virus origins and receptor binding. The Lancet. 2020;395(10224):565-74.

[36] Boni M, Lemey P, Jiang X, Lam T, Perry B, Castoe T, et al. Evolutionary origins of the SARS-CoV-2 sarbecovirus lineage responsible for the COVID-19 pandemic. Nat Microbiol. Nature Publishing Group; 2020.

[37] Zhang Y. Initial genome release of novel coronavirus. 2020.

[38] COVID TC, Team R. Severe Outcomes Among Patients with Coronavirus Disease 2019 (COVID-19)-United States, February 12–March 16, 2020. MMWR Morb Mortal Wkly Rep. 2020;69(12):343-6.

[39] COVID W. strategy update. April, 14, 2020.

[40] AmericanWell. Telehealth Index: 2019 Consumer Survey 2019 [cited 2020 December 14th]. Available from: https://static.americanwell.com/app/uploads/2019/07/American-Well-Telehealth-Index-2019-Consumer-Survey-eBook2.pdf.

[41] Alexander GC, Tajanlangit M, Heyward J, Mansour O, Qato DM, Stafford RS. Use and Content of Primary Care Office-Based vs Telemedicine Care Visits During the COVID-19 Pandemic in the US. JAMA Network Open. 2020;3(10):e2021476-e.

[42] Papautsky EL, Hamlish T. Patient-reported treatment delays in breast cancer care during the COVID-19 pandemic. Breast cancer research and treatment. 2020;184(1):249-54.

[43] Dai M, Liu D, Liu M, Zhou F, Li G, Chen Z, et al. Patients with cancer appear more vulnerable to SARS-CoV-2: a multicenter study during the COVID-19 outbreak. Cancer Discov 10 (6): 783-791. 2020.

[44] Wang H, Zhang L. Risk of COVID-19 for patients with cancer. The Lancet Oncology. 2020;21(4):e181.

[45] Xia Y, Jin R, Zhao J, Li W, Shen H. Risk of COVID-19 for cancer patients. Lancet Oncol. 2020;21(4).

[46] Kamboj M, Sepkowitz KA. Nosocomial infections in patients with cancer. The lancet oncology. 2009;10(6):589-97.

[47] Li J-Y, Duan X-F, Wang L-P, Xu Y-J, Huang L, Zhang T-F, et al. Selective depletion of regulatory T cell subsets by docetaxel treatment in patients with nonsmall cell lung cancer. Journal of immunology research. 2014;2014.

[48] Longbottom ER, Torrance HD, Owen HC, Fragkou PC, Hinds CJ, Pearse RM, et al. Features of postoperative immune suppression are reversible with interferon gamma and independent of interleukin-6 pathways. Annals of surgery. 2016;264(2):370-7.

[49] Sica A, Massarotti M. Myeloid suppressor cells in cancer and autoimmunity. Journal of autoimmunity. 2017;85:117-25.

[50] Liang W, Guan W, Chen R, Wang W, Li J, Xu K, et al. Cancer patients in SARS-CoV-2 infection: a nationwide analysis in China. The Lancet Oncology. 2020; 21(3):335-7.

[51] Miyashita H, Mikami T, Chopra N, Yamada T, Chernyavsky S, Rizk D, et al. Do patients with cancer have a poorer prognosis of COVID-19? An experience in New York City. Annals of Oncology. 2020.

[52] States CfDCaPCitU. People with Certain Medical Conditions: CDC; 2020 [Available from: https://www.cdc.gov/coronavirus/2019-ncov/need-extra-precautions/people-with-medical-conditions.html.

[53] Gupta S, Hayek S, Wang W, Investigators S-C. Factors associated with death in critically Ill patients with coronavirus disease 2019 in the US. JAMA Intern Med. 2020: e203596. 2020.

[54] Kuderer NM, Choueiri TK, Shah DP, Shyr Y, Rubinstein SM, Rivera DR, et al. Clinical impact of COVID-19 on patients with cancer (CCC19): a cohort study. The Lancet. 2020.

[55] Emens LA. Breast cancer immunobiology driving immunotherapy: vaccines and immune checkpoint blockade. Expert review of anticancer therapy. 2012;12(12):1597-611.

[56] Kristensen VN, Vaske CJ, Ursini-Siegel J, Van Loo P, Nordgard SH, Sachidanandam R, et al. Integrated molecular profiles of invasive breast tumors and ductal carcinoma in situ (DCIS) reveal differential vascular and interleukin signaling. Proceedings of the National Academy of Sciences. 2012;109(8):2802-7.

[57] DeNardo DG, Barreto JB, Andreu P, Vasquez L, Tawfik D, Kolhatkar N, et al. CD4+ T cells regulate pulmonary metastasis of mammary carcinomas by enhancing protumor properties of macrophages. Cancer cell. 2009;16(2):91-102.

[58] Miller K, Siegel R, Jemal A. Cancer treatment & survivorship facts & figures 2016-2017. Atlanta: American Cancer Society. 2016.

[59] Mackall C, Fleisher T, Brown M, Magrath I, Shad A, Horowitz M, et al. Lymphocyte depletion during treatment with intensive chemotherapy for cancer. Blood. 1994;84(7):2221-8.

[60] Strender LE, Blomgren H, Petrini B, Wasserman J, Forsgren M, Norberg R, et al. Immunologic monitoring in breast cancer patients receiving postoperative adjuvant chemotherapy. Cancer. 1981;48(9):1996-2002.

[61] Brunvand MW, Collins C, Livingston RB, Raghu G. Pneumocystis carinii pneumonia associated with profound lymphopenia and abnormal T-lymphocyte subset ratios during treatment for early-stage breast carcinoma. Cancer. 1991;67(9):2407-9.

[62] Gaynor N, Crown J, Collins DM, editors. Immune checkpoint inhibitors: Key trials and an emerging role in breast

cancer. Seminars in cancer biology; 2020: Elsevier.

[63] Planes-Laine G, Rochigneux P, Bertucci F, Chrétien A-S, Viens P, Sabatier R, et al. PD-1/PD-L1 targeting in breast cancer: the first clinical evidences are emerging—a literature review. Cancers. 2019;11(7):1033.

[64] Rossi E, Schinzari G, Tortora G. Pneumonitis from immune checkpoint inhibitors and COVID-19: current concern in cancer treatment. Journal for Immunotherapy of Cancer. 2020;8(2).

[65] Wang DY, Salem J-E, Cohen JV, Chandra S, Menzer C, Ye F, et al. Fatal toxic effects associated with immune checkpoint inhibitors: a systematic review and meta-analysis. JAMA oncology. 2018;4(12):1721-8.

[66] Whitfield SJ, Taylor C, Risdall JE, Griffiths GD, Jones JT, Williamson ED, et al. Interference of the T cell and antigen-presenting cell costimulatory pathway using CTLA4-Ig (abatacept) prevents Staphylococcal enterotoxin B pathology. The Journal of Immunology. 2017;198(10):3989-98.

[67] Saha B, Jaklic B, Harlan DM, Gray GS, June CH, Abe R. Toxic shock syndrome toxin-1-induced death is prevented by CTLA4Ig. The Journal of Immunology. 1996;157(9):3869-75.

[68] Schönrich G, Raftery MJ. The PD-1/PD-L1 axis and virus infections: a delicate balance. Frontiers in cellular and infection microbiology. 2019;9:207.

[69] Diao B, Wang C, Tan Y, Chen X, Liu Y, Ning L, et al. Reduction and functional exhaustion of T cells in patients with coronavirus disease 2019 (COVID-19). Frontiers in Immunology. 2020;11:827.

[70] Cortese I, Muranski P, Enose-Akahata Y, Ha S-K, Smith B, Monaco M, et al. Pembrolizumabtreatmentforprogressive multifocal leukoencephalopathy. New England Journal of Medicine. 2019;380(17):1597-605.

[71] Shah KP, Song H, Ye F, Moslehi JJ, Balko JM, Salem J-E, et al. Demographic Factors Associated with Toxicity in Patients Treated with Anti–Programmed Cell Death-1 Therapy. Cancer immunology research. 2020;8(7):851-5.

[72] Awadalla M, Golden DLA, Mahmood SS, Alvi RM, Mercaldo ND, Hassan MZ, et al. Influenza vaccination and myocarditis among patients receiving immune checkpoint inhibitors. Journal for immunotherapy of cancer. 2019;7(1):53.

[73] Polk A, Svane I-M, Andersson M, Nielsen D. Checkpoint inhibitors in breast cancer–current status. Cancer treatment reviews. 2018;63:122-34.

[74] Miller KD, Siegel RL, Lin CC, Mariotto AB, Kramer JL, Rowland JH, et al. Cancer treatment and survivorship statistics, 2016. CA: a cancer journal for clinicians. 2016;66(4):271-89.

[75] Verma R, Foster RE, Horgan K, Mounsey K, Nixon H, Smalle N, et al. Lymphocyte depletion and repopulation after chemotherapy for primary breast cancer. Breast Cancer Research. 2016;18(1):10.

[76] Formenti SC, Demaria S. Systemic effects of local radiotherapy. The lancet oncology. 2009;10(7):718-26.

[77] Kang D-H, Weaver MT, Park N-J, Smith B, McArdle T, Carpenter J. Significant impairment in immune recovery following cancer treatment. Nursing research. 2009;58(2):105.

[78] Colzani E, Johansson AL, Liljegren A, Foukakis T, Clements M, Adolfsson J, et al. Time-dependent risk of developing distant metastasis in breast cancer patients according to treatment, age and tumour characteristics. British journal of cancer. 2014;110(5):1378-84.

[79] McCarthy CM, Mehrara BJ, Riedel E, Davidge K, Hinson A, Disa JJ, et al. Predicting complications following expander/implant breast reconstruction: an outcomes analysis based on preoperative clinical risk. Plastic and reconstructive surgery. 2008;121(6):1886-92.

[80] Benveniste MF, Gomez D, Carter BW, Betancourt Cuellar SL, Shroff GS, Benveniste APA, et al. Recognizing Radiation Therapy-related Complications in the Chest. Radiographics : a review publication of the Radiological Society of North America, Inc. 2019;39(2):344-66.

[81] Almuwaqqat Z, Meisel JL, Barac A, Parashar S. Breast Cancer and Heart Failure. Heart failure clinics. 2019;15(1):65-75.

[82] Morarji K, McArdle O, Hui K, Gingras-Hill G, Ahmed S, Greenblatt EM, et al. Ovarian function after chemotherapy in young breast cancer survivors. Curr Oncol. 2017;24(6):e494-e502.

[83] Schaapveld M, Visser O, Louwman MJ, de Vries EG, Willemse PH, Otter R, et al. Risk of new primary nonbreast cancers after breast cancer treatment: a Dutch population-based study. Journal of clinical oncology : official journal of the American Society of Clinical Oncology. 2008;26(8):1239-46.

[84] Pinquart M, Duberstein PR. Associations of social networks with cancer mortality: a meta-analysis. Crit Rev Oncol Hematol. 2010;75(2):122-37.

[85] Strasser F, Sweeney C, Willey J, Benisch-Tolley S, Palmer JL, Bruera E. Impact of a half-day multidisciplinary symptom control and palliative care outpatient clinic in a comprehensive cancer center on recommendations, symptom intensity, and patient satisfaction: a retrospective descriptive study. J Pain Symptom Manage. 2004;27(6):481-91.

[86] Carlson LE, Bultz BD. Efficacy and medical cost offset of psychosocial interventions in cancer care: making the case for economic analyses. Psychooncology. 2004;13(12):837-49; discussion 50-6.

[87] Holland JC. American Cancer Society Award lecture. Psychological care of patients: psycho-oncology's contribution. J Clin Oncol. 2003;21(23 Suppl):253s–65s.

[88] Elimimian EB, Elson L, Stone E, Butler RS, Doll M, Roshon S, et al. A pilot study of improved psychological distress with art therapy in patients with cancer undergoing chemotherapy. BMC Cancer. 2020;20(1):899.

[89] Applebaum AJ, Stein EM, Lord-Bessen J, Pessin H, Rosenfeld B, Breitbart W. Optimism, social support, and mental health outcomes in patients with advanced cancer. Psycho-oncology. 2014;23(3):299-306.

[90] Waters EA, Liu Y, Schootman M, Jeffe DB. Worry about cancer progression and low perceived social support: implications for quality of life among early-stage breast cancer patients. Ann Behav Med. 2013;45(1):57-68.

[91] Kroenke CH, Kwan ML, Neugut AI, Ergas IJ, Wright JD, Caan BJ, et al. Social

networks, social support mechanisms, and quality of life after breast cancer diagnosis. Breast Cancer Res Tr. 2013;139(2):515-27.

[92] Bitonte RA, De Santo M. Art Therapy: An Underutilized, yet Effective Tool. Ment Illn. 2014;6(1):5354-.

Chapter 9

Implication of Connexin 43 as a Tumor Suppressor in Pathogenesis of Breast Cancer

Rabiya Rashid, Shazia Ali and Mahboob-Ul-Hussain

Abstract

Breast cancer (BC) is a global public health burden, constituting the highest cancer incidence in women worldwide. Connexins 43 proteins propagate intercellular communication, gap junction intercellular communication (GJIC), remarkably expressed in several tumor types including liver, prostate, and breast. This domain of Cx43 possesses functionally critical sites identical to those involved in gating of channel and phosphorylation sites for various kinases. However, the mechanism by which Cx43 down regulation occurs in breast cancer is far from clear. Several mechanisms like Cx43 promoter hyper-methylation or a cancer-specific reduction of Cx43 expression/trafficking by the modulation of various components of the Cx43 life cycle give the idea to be involved in the down regulation of Connexins in mammary glands, but irreversible mutational alterations have not yet been proved to be among them. Summarily, the efficacy or specificity of these drugs can be increased by a combinatory approach considering an effect on both the Connexins and their regulatory molecules. This chapter will summarize the knowledge about the connexins and gap junction activities in breast cancer highlighting the differential expression and functional dynamics of connexins in the pathogenesis of the disease.

Keywords: Breast Cancer, Connexin, Tumor Suppressor, Gap junction, mammary gland

1. Introduction

Cancers that originate from the breast tissue are called as Breast cancers. Quite often, these cancers originate from the epithelial cells lining the milk ducts or lobules supplying the ducts with milk [1]. Sub-classification of breast cancer into various types is done on the basis of certain characteristics that the cancers develop depending on their origin i.e. whether cancer originates from glandular portion or ductal portion of the breast. Accordingly, cancers that stem from lobules are called as lobular carcinomas, whereas those stemming from ducts are called as ductal carcinomas. Once Primary tumors become invasive, it spreads beyond its place of origin (Breast) to the regional lymph nodes. It may also metastasize i.e., expand to different organ systems of the body, thereby becoming systemic in nature. On the basis of this expansion, breast cancer is of two types Non-invasive or in-situ and invasive. A non-invasive or in-situ cancer is one where the cancer cells remain confined to boundaries of the lobular unit or draining duct of their origin. On the other hand, cancer cells that traverse outside the basement membrane of the lobules or ducts into the surrounding normal tissues are classified as invasive cancers. Apart from these, there are other types of breast cancer with different stages, varied aggressiveness and different genetic makeup. These factors greatly affect the chances of survival of a patient. Several breast cancers are up regulated by estrogens. These cancer cells carry estrogen receptors on their surfaces and are called Estrogen Receptor-positive cancers or ER-positive cancers. Similarly, some women suffer from another type of breast cancer called as HER2-positive breast cancer. HER2 is a gene responsible for cell growth, division and repair. Increased copy number of HER2 gene may result in faster growth of cancers. Women with HER2-positive breast cancer have higher incidence of disease recurrence making it as a risk factor for breast cancer recurrence. The disease is also more aggressive than women who do not have this type of breast cancer.

2. Stages of breast cancer

Expansion of a cancer determines its stage. Stages of a cancer indicate whether the cancer is limited to the area of origin or has spread to other healthy tissues of the body. Four important characteristics determine a cancer stage:

a. Size of the cancer.

b. Type of cancer i.e. invasive or non-invasive.

c. Has cancer reached lymph nodes,

d. Has cancer metastasized to other body parts.

Firstly, on the basis of extent of the cancer, it can be classified as local, regional or distant. A cancer is **local,** when it is confined within the breast (where it originated). It is **regional** when lymph nodes are involved. And it is **distant** when it has metastasized to other body parts as well.

There is another staging system used to describe the cancer called as TNM staging system. The TNM System is based on three components - size of the tumor (denoted by T), involvement of the lymph node (denoted by N) and whether the cancer has metastasized (denoted by M).

Stage 0: It is a non-invasive stage, during this stage cancer is present at its origin e.g., Ductal Carcinoma In Situ (DCIS). There is no indication of the cancer cells or non-cancerous abnormal cells traveling beyond their origin to neighboring normal tissues.

Stage I: This stage describes an invasive breast cancer i.e., cancer cells invade neighboring normal tissues. There are chances of microscopic invasion in this stage. In such an invasion, the cancer cells have just begun to travel outside the boundaries of their duct or lobule. However, the invading cancer cells are not more than 1 mm.

Stage II: This stage is further sub-categorized into stages IIA and IIB, both describing a different invasive breast cancer. Stage IIA refers to an invasive breast cancer where the tumor cannot be located in the breast but lymph nodes (axillary) under the arm show presence of cancer cells.

Stage IIB: Refers to an invasive breast cancer where a tumor sized between 2 cm and 5 cm has spread to axillary lymph nodes.

Stage III: This stage is further sub-categorized into three stages - Stages IIIA, IIIB and IIIC. Stage IIIA refers to an invasive breast cancer where either the tumor cannot be located in the breast but cancer is found in axillary lymph nodes which are clumped or clinged to other structures, or lymph nodes at breast bone may be involved too.

Stage IIIB: Defines an invasive breast cancer stage where cancer has involved chest wall or breast skin or both and may involve axillary lymph nodes and showing Stage IIIA like features too.

Stage IIIC: Refers to an invasive breast cancer where there is no evidence of cancer in the breast or, in the event there exists a tumor, it is of any size, which may be involving chest wall or breast skin, or both. In this stage, the cancer has also extended to the lymph nodes below or above the collarbone and may also have spread to axillary lymph nodes or to lymph nodes near the breastbone.

Stage IV: This stage describes an invasive breast cancer which has extended outside the breast and adjacent lymph nodes and has affected other organs of the body e.g., lungs, bones, brain, liver, skin etc.

3. Epidemiology of breast cancer

In Modern world, occurrence of non-communicable diseases is increasing day by day [2, 3]. This is mainly due to factors like increased lifespan, prolonged exposure to risk factors and changes in lifestyle. While being one of the most crucial diseases in the world, cancer is also regarded as a complicated-on account of being multi-factorial, epidemiologically. In 2012 alone, around 14.9 million new cases of cancer were tradition, culture, food habits, intra-community marriages and ethnicity. In recent past recorded. It is estimated that in the next two decades, this number will be around 22 million [4]. Now a day, breast cancer is becoming more common in women and is cosmopolitan in nature with high rate of incidence [5]. It accounts for 25% of all types of cancers, recording 1.7 million new cases per year. It is also the second common most cancer [4]. As per WHO, the latest incidence rate of breast cancer in east Africa to west Europe ranges from 19.4 to 89.7 per one lakh people respectively [6]. Other than its fast growth rate in South America and Africa, breast cancer incidence in on rise in several Asian countries too. For instance, Japan witnessed a 6% increase per year from 1999 to 2008. In Australia, mortality rate due to breast cancer has reduced by 2%. While it is increasing in several countries. Malaysia and Thailand recorded the highest increase. The ratio of mortality and incidence of breast cancer in the world and Asia-Pacific countries is 0.30 and 0.27 respectively. However, this ratio of mortality and breast cancer incidence is 0.2 and 0.41 in the Pacific and Southeast-Asian countries respectively [7]. Not so long ago, breast cancer incidence was rare in South Korea. However, now, the incidence and death rate from breast cancer has increased [8]. Hong Kong has seen a decline in the incidence [9]. Generally, different regions show different breast cancer incidence due to difference in risk factors, level of education, different life expectancy, screening programs [10], and cancer registration [2]. The number of diagnosed breast cancer cases is increasing because of the increased life expectancy and increased full health screens [10]. Cancer accounts for around 3–4 million deaths worldwide annually. Of these, 2–3 million deaths occur in developing countries [11]. In India, cervical cancer has a higher occurrence than breast cancer. On the contrary, our state (J&K) in the Indian Subcontinent, Kashmir shows a reverse trend (World Health Organization, 1978) (**Figure 1**). Rise in breast cancer in Kashmir valley is considered a major health concern. Experts attribute this increase in breast cancer to various factors like sedentary lifestyle, bottle feeding, late

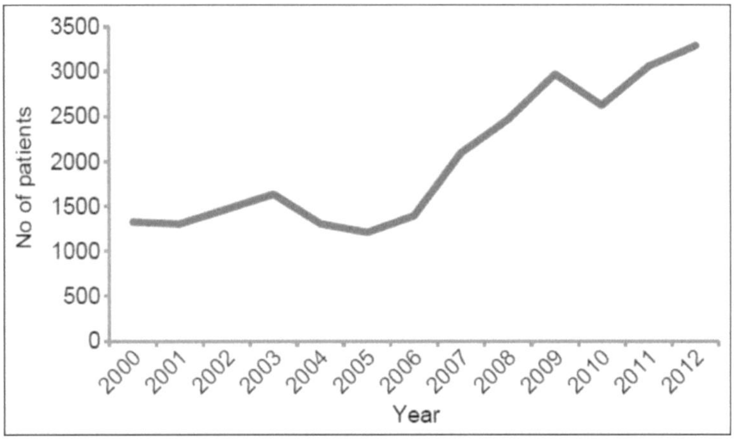

Figure 1.
Shows year-wise number of registered cancer patients, incidence sites and cancer trends 2000–2012). Adapted from Wani [12].

marriages etc. Kashmir valley is quite different from other areas with respect to its unique geographical location, Kashmir has seen a huge increase in the occurrence of breast cancer among its unexplored ethnic population. The overall cancer incidence in Kashmir region is increasing. In men, esophagus and gastroesophageal (GE) junction, lung, stomach, colon, rectum, lymph nodes, skin, laryngopharynx, blood, prostate and brain are the common sites of cancer. While in females the common sites are breast, esophagus and GE junction, ovary, colon, rectum, stomach, lung, gallbladder, lymph nodes, blood and brain.

4. Connexin 43 and breast cancer

Connexin 43 is the most widely expressed gap-junction protein in normal breast tissue and is thought to play important role in normal mammogenesis, lactogenesis and involution [13]. Cx43 is not expressed in normal breast stem cells but is expressed in the normal breast epithelial cells derived from these breast stem cells [14–16]. Studies have shown that Cx43 is down regulated at the mRNA and protein level in human breast tumors and several human mammary tumor cell lines [17]. Decreased expression of connexin gap junctions is seen in breast cancer at various stages of progression and restoration of gap-junction intercellular communication. Studies have shown that Cx43 is down regulated at the mRNA and protein level in human breast tumors and several human mammary tumor cell lines [17]. Decreased expression of connexin gap junctions is seen in breast cancer at various stages of progression and restoration of gap-junction intercellular communication. Under in vitro conditions it has been seen that the upregulation of connexins restore normal phenotype and reduce tumor growth in vivo conditions [18, 19]. Various studies have shown that down-regulation of Cx43 plays role in primary tumor formation as well as its metastasis in breast tissue. Primary breast cancer is generally composed of tumor cells and surrounding connective tissue. The arrangement within cancer creates multiple patterns of cell–cell interactions among tumor cells and between tumor cells and normal neighboring stromal cells. Among, these patterns the GJIC involving Cx43 is considered to be initial step associated with malignant cell transformation. Studies have shown down-regulation of Connexin 43 gap-junction occurs in human breast cancer tissues compared with the non-neoplastic breast tissue surrounding primary tissue. It has been seen that re-expression of Cx43 reverses the malignancy of human mammary carcinoma cells [19–21]. In, rat mammary carcinoma induced by DMBA data obtained demonstrates that connexin 43 gap junction loss is a common feature of transformed mammary neoplastic cells. Furthermore, data obtained with rat mammary carcinoma, induced by DMBA also demonstrates that the loss of connexin 43 gap junction is a common feature of mammary neoplastic transformed cells. In human mammary carcinoma (MDA-MB-435) cells it has observed that the Cx43 re-expression suppresses the cancer phenotype, increases ability of cells to differentiate into well defined 3D structures and also reduces the tumor growth in animal models [20, 22]. Studies have also shown that down-regulation of endogenous connexin 43 expression by small interfering RNA promoted a more aggressive phenotype in human breast cancer cell lines. It was seen in this study that Cx43 reduced the expression of fibroblastic factor receptor (FGFR) and of other proteins that are involved in tumor progression. Studies have revealed that over expression of Cx43 in tumor cells not only restores growth control, but they also revert to less malignant phenotypes [18]. Upregulation of Cx43 by the drugs like genistein and quercetin leads to GJIC-independent inhibition of cell proliferation [23]. Cx43 plays role in tumorigenesis probably by inhibiting angiogenesis independently of cell communication as inhibition of Cx43 expression by RNAi in breast cancer Hs578t cells, resulted in faster growth and increased aggressiveness of the cells, TSP-1 expression was reduced while pro-angiogenic factor VEGF was upregulated. Similar results were observed in MDA-MB-231 cells over expressing Cx43. In addition conditioned media from these cells inhibited in vitro endothelial cell tubulogenesis and migration [24]. Additionally, tumor angiogenesis was decreased in xenografts of Cx43-overexpressing MDA-MB-231 cells. Altogether these findings suggest that Cx43 plays tumor suppressing role by mediating cell proliferation, migration and angiogenesis, enduring support to relatedness between physiological variation in Cx43 levels and aggressive of breast cancer. Tumor metastasis, a multi-step process involves the entry of transformed cells into the circulation after dissociating from the site of origin, extravasation from the vascular system and proliferation into tumor masses at secondary tissue sites. Different stages of this metastatic cascade depend both on cell–cell and cell-matrix interactions [25]. Metastasis has been shown to be promoted by down-regulation of connexins as the breast metastasis suppressor 1 gene exogenous expression in MDA-MB-435 cells led to upregulation of Cx43 and restoration of GJIC, providing evidence that connexins act as tumor suppressors in metastasis [26]. The migratory potential and ability to invade through basement membrane matrix was found to diminish in cells with exogenous expression of Cx26 and Cx43 during functional in vitro studies [27] along with a slight drop-off in matrix metalloproteinase activity [28]. Additionally, studies show decrease in the number of metastases to lungs in mice injected with breast cancer cells expressing Cx43 relative to mice injected with vector controls only [20]. The movement of cancer cells across the endothelial cell barrier as they move in and out of the blood vessels has been shown to be a key step in metastasis and studies have shown that Connexins play an important role in tumor cell vascular intravasation and extravasation [29]. Co-culturing of endothelial cells with breast cancer cells results in the reduction of GJIC in endothelial cells. This reduction weakens cell–cell contacts and also it becomes easier for cells to cross endothelial barrier during the process of extravasation and intravasation [30]. This fact was supported by another study which shows that over expression of Cx43 in HBL-100 breast cancer cells (GJIC deficient) makes them capable of forming heterocellular junctions. These junctions allow dye transfer between human microvascular endothelial cell expressing cx43 and breast cancer cells resulting in tumor cell diapedesis. Treatment of endothelial culture with GJIC inhibitors or co culturing of endothelial cells with breast cancer cells that express mutated or non-functional Cx43 results in blockage of trans endothelial migration [31]. Hence these studies imply that both homocellular GJIC between endothelial cells and heterocellular GJIC between endothelial cells and breast cancer cells facilitate trans endothelial migration. A series of studies performed on the effects of metastatic breast cancer cells on osteoblast differentiation with MDA-MB-231 and MC3T3-E1 cells showed inhibition of osteoblast differentiation by conditioned medium from breast cancer cells [32, 33]. It has also been demonstrated by other studies that in MDA-MB-231 Cx43 expression results in decreased expression of OB-cadherin [34] a similar trend was also found in Cx43 expressing MDA-MB-435 cells. Decrease in the expression of N-cadherin, a protein which is involved in increased motility, invasion and metastases of breast cancer cells [35, 36] has been observed in in Cx43 over expressing MDA-MB-231 cells [34] this clearly shows that it contributes to decreased metastasis in vivo. In human glioblastoma cells it has been seen that Cx43 enhances response to chemotherapeutic agents or low serum hence confirming the fact that Cx43 shows anti metastatic effect [37]. In human breast cancer tissue, studies have also demonstrated that expression of Cx43 is directly correlated with the expression of BAK (Bcl-2 homologous antagonist/killer), a pro-apoptotic gene of the Bcl-2 family [38]. In human mammary carcinoma cell, MDA-MB-435 Cx43 suppressed the cancer phenotype and cell growth in culture and in animal models. There remains little doubt that down regulation of Cx43 plays a very important role in the primary tumor formation and its metastasis in mammary glands. However, the mechanism by which Cx43 down regulation occurs in breast cancer is far from clear. Several mechanisms like Cx43 promoter hyper-methylation or a cancer-specific reduction of Cx43 expression/trafficking by the modulation of various components of the Cx43 life cycle appear to be involved in the down regulation of Connexins in mammary glands, but irreversible mutational alterations have not yet been proved to be among them. Therefore, the role of Cx43 in carcinogenesis requires further investigations. Additional studies on Cx43 in different cancers, thus, will establish its role in cancer signaling and thus as a therapeutic target.

5. Regulation of Connexin 43 by epigenetic mechanisms and transcription factors

Tumors and transformed cell lines generally exhibit down regulation of Connexin expression. This down regulation is said to be responsible for the loss of proliferating control. However, deletion or mutation of connexin gene as a common factor in human tumors has not yet been demonstrated by various intensive studies on the subject. On the other hand, what various studies have shown is that silencing of Connexin expression in several kinds of malignant cells can be caused due to epigenetic inactivation of the promoter region by hypermethylation. Studies have also indicated that types of cells and connexins determine the effects of DNA methyltransferase inhibitors on connexin expression, as illustrated by Vinekn et al. in a review [39]. A correlation was established with micrometastasis into lymph nodes and the lack of Cx43 mRNA expression in adjacent normal lung cancer tissue in human non-small lung cancers [40]. Patients lacking Cx43 mRNA possessed higher frequency of promoter methylation compared with Cx43 mRNA-positive patients, as reported by Chen. Their data also indicates a possible interference of promoter methylation with AP-1 binding to the promoter which results in lack of Cx43 gene expression. The human Cx43 proximal promoters possesses several binding sides for Sp1 and AP1 transcription factors and have been demonstrated to be indispensable for optimal promoter activity by promoter/report assays and

Sp1/AP1 over expression studies. The Sp1- and Ap1- binding sites were shown to contribute to the activity of the promoter. Each of them also contributed to bind the transcription factors Sp1/Sp3 or AP1, respectively. Both Sp1 and Sp3 resulted in the rat Cx43 promoter activation during trans-activation assays. These findings indicate the importance of the transcription factors Sp1, Sp3 and AP1 in rat Cx43 proximal promoter activity. Cell type-specific expression of Cx43 may thus depend on additional activators or repressors in different Cx43-expressing cell types (including cardiomyocytes) as similarities exist in proximal promoter regulation by universally expressed transcription factors (Sp1, Sp3, AP1). Although the mechanism Connexin gene silencing by DNA methylation is clear, the origin of this epigenetic modification still remains elusive. In liver cancer, elevated DNMT1 mRNA levels are thought to decrease expression of connexins, in casu Cx26 [41]. Moreover, the aberrant binding of transcription factors to methylated Connexin gene promoters may contribute to poor Connexin expression in cancer cells. This is supported by the decreased Cx43 gene transcription accompanied by DNA methylation in human non-small cell lung cancer cells. The decreased Cx43 gene transcription is also correlated with reduced binding of activator protein 1 (AP1) to its promoter [40]. Furthermore, in human breast cancer cells [42] and rat liver cancer cells [43] the Sp1 cis-acting elements of the Cx26 and the Cx32 gene promoter are especially rich in methylated CpG dinucleotides.

6. Regulation of Connexin 43 by micro RNAs

Almost one-tenth of all new cancers and 23% of cancer cases detected in females are breast carcinomas with more than 1 million diagnoses every year worldwide [44, 45]. Major causes of this disease-related death are relapse and metastasis [46, 47]. Recent studies that on the metastatic mechanisms of breast cancer suggest the gap junction to be a major regulator of tumor metastasis [48]. Located at the cell membrane, the gap junction primarily comprises of different connexin proteins. These connexin proteins are closely associated with numerous functions of the cell [49, 50]. Connexins constitute a family of 21 members with Cx43 being abundantly expressed in the mammary gland [49]. It is reported that Cx43 plays an important role in normal cell migration [51] and tumor cell invasion [52]. As such, promising strategies in regulating cell functions are provided by the regulation of Cx43 expression [53, 54]. Different transcription factors tightly regulate the expression of CX43 gene at transcription level. Studies have found that Sp1 (specificity protein 1), Sp3, AP-1 (activating protein 1) and c-Jun can promote transcriptional activity of Cx43 gene by directly binding to its promoter [55, 54] addition, at the post-transcription level Cx43 is also closely regulated by miRNAs [53, 56, 57]. miRNAs, largest groups of posttranscriptional regulators, [58]. Eight bases at the 5′end of miRNAs, are involved in posttranscriptional regulation. These two to eight bases could bind to the 3′-UTR of the target genes in order to bring about inhibition of gene expression at mRNA level [58]. By virtue of their direct or indirect regulation of target gene expression, miRNAs regulate a number of biological processes. The processes include cell cycle [59], growth [60], apoptosis [60], differentiation [61] and stress reaction [62]. Studies have identified miR-1, miR-206, and miR-381 as potent suppressors of Cx43 [53, 56, 63]. Cx43 has been found to enhance metastasis in breast cancer cells. It has been proven to be a direct negative target for miR-206, miR-1 and miR-133 and an indirect target for miR 381 [8]. During the myoblast differentiation in vitro and in vivo, two related miRNAs, miR-206 and miR-1, cause inhibition of Cx43 protein expression without altering Cx43 mRNA levels [63]. Further it has been reported by Anderson et al. that Cx43 mRNA contains two binding sites in its 3'UTR for miR-206/miR-1, both of which are essential for an efficient down regulation. Also, they observed sections of eight nucleotides in the 3'UTR of Cx43 gene that are complementary to the first eight nucleotides from the 5′ end of miR-1. Which then they proved that miR-1 binds to these nucleotide sequences. miR-1 was also shown to cause reduction of Cx43 levels in isolated neonatal rat ventricular myocytes in culture [64]. They further found two putative target sequences in the 3′ UTR of Cx43 for miR-206 and proved that miR-206 that is expressed ectopically binds these sites. Moreover, the ectopic expression of miR-206 downregulated the endogenous expression Cx43 gene without affecting Cx43 mRNA expression. The continuous expression of miR-206 in osteoblasts resulted in decreased expression of osteoblast differentiation and Cx43 protein expression. The suppression of Cx43 gene expression was caused by miR-381 via the promoter region −500/−250 miR-381 could directly bind the sequences CACUUGUAU in the 3′UTR. Site-directed gene mutation was done (CCAAT/enhancer-binding protein α) in order to inhibit C/EBPα expression. By binding it to a canonic element (AATTGTC) located at −459/−453 in the promoter region of the Cx43 gene, they identified C/EBPα as a novel transcription factor. Therefore, miR-381 causes C/EBPα dependent Cx43 suppression in breast cancer cells.

7. IRES mediated regulation of Connexin 43

Connexin 43 (Cx43) is one of the main gap junction (cell–cell channel) proteins expressed in the heart ventricle. Constitutive expression of Connexin 43 has been found to be responsible for the anisotropic propagation of action potentials in the heart [65]. And also, Cx43 gap junctions are essential for the synchronous contraction of the myometrium of the uterus during labour pain. While the expression of Cx43 is ordinarily sparse in the myometrium, the ovarian hormones and mechanical stretch upregulate it [66]. This upregulation is seen at the transcriptional as well as the translational level, as there is accumulation of Cx43 mRNA before the swift advent of Cx43 protein, just prior to childbirth [67–70]. The Cx43 gene like most of the connexin genes consists of two exons separated by a large intron. Exon 1 contains most of the 5P-untranslated region (5P-Utr) while the remaining 13 bases of the 5P-UTR followed by the entire coding region and the 3P-UTR are contained in Exon 2. There is wide acceptance of observation that in eukaryotes, protein synthesis initiation begins with the binding of the small ribosomal subunit to the 5P-cap structure. Then the mRNA is scanned by the 40S ribosome until it encounters an AUG codon where the 60S ribosomal subunit joins, and hence the translation begins. Between the cap structure and the first AUG codon, most cellular mRNAs contain fewer than 50 nt between the cap structure and the first AUG codon but the 5P-UTR of Cx43 mRNA has been found to 208 nt. In addition, the 5P-UTR of Cx43 mRNA has a stable secondary structure. The scanning of the 40S ribosome can be inhibited by such structures. The secondary structures of the Cx43 IRES and most of the other described IRES elements have a semi-conserved Y-like structure, which is suggested to have role in the IRES mediated translation in eukaryotic cells in Stress conditions. Inhibition of cap-dependent translation is one of the cellular responses to stress [71]. This inhibition allows continuation of synthesis of proteins essential for survival and stops the synthesis of non-essential proteins. Illustrations for this are as follows: VEGF is translated in response to hypoxia [72], the translation of the chaperone proteins Bip [73] and hsp70 takes place under conditions of cellular stress in response to misfolded and degraded proteins and in the infarcted myocardium FGF-2 functions in the salvage of cells [74]. In all these genes, IRES elements have been found that are translated even under stress conditions. The need is to maintain intercellular communication via Cx43 channels even under certain stressful conditions likely. For instance, in the hypoxic hear gap junctional remodeling occurs [75] requiring the synthesis of new Cx43. Recent reports have claimed that in addition to estrogen, mechanical stretch is required to upregulate expression of Cx43 in the uterus at the commencement of labor [66]. The fetus grows faster than the uterus during the later phase of pregnancy which causes physical stretch in the myometrium. As such, Cx43 must be speedily upregulated during this time. A mechanism by which a high level of translation can be accomplished during this stress may be offered by the IRES.

8. Carboxy terminal domain of Connexin 43 and human breast cancer

Cellular communication is paramount for tissue/organ homeostasis in multicellular organisms. Exchange of small ions, secondary messengers and small metabolites required for electrical and bio-chemical coupling between cells is mediated via intercellular channels known as gap junctions [76, 77]. Each gap junction is formed by association of Connexin proteins. Human genome contains 21 different Connexin genes, expressed differentially in various types of cells and tissues [78]. Among these gap junction proteins, connexin 43 (Cx43) is major gap junction protein which is widely expressed across tissues and besides its role in mediating cell to cell communication, it also plays very critical role in cellular proliferation [79]. More precisely, Cx43 acts a tumor suppressor [80] usually downregulated in various diseases such as cancer [81, 82], connexin 43 possesses long cytosolic C-terminus and most of the non-canonical functions of connexin 43 are attributed to it [83] (**Figure 2**).

More interestingly independent of full length Cx43, CT-Cx43 expression has been found to occur in various cell types [85]. This CT domain is subjected to various post translational modifications like phosphorylation, S nitrosylation and

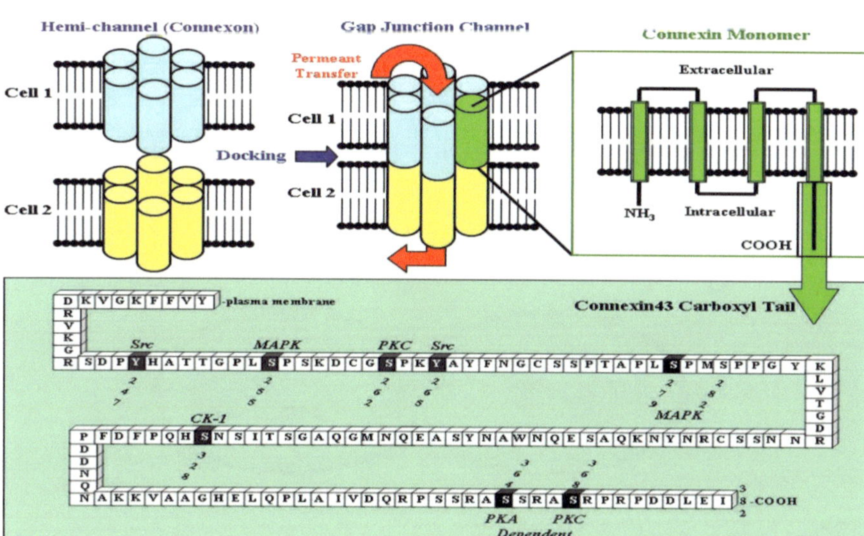

Figure 2.
Gap junctional intercellular communication (GJC) mediated by connexin proteins. Hexameric arrangements of connexin monomers comprise a hemi-channel or connexon. Adjoining cells each contribute one connexon to form a complete gap junction channel. For several connexin types, the assembly, gating and turnover of this channel are regulated to a large extent via phosphorylation of the cytoplasmic tail by various cellular kinases including: Src, PKC and MAPK. Adapted from (king and Bertram, 2005) [84].

truncation [86]. Also CT-Cx43 has been shown to interact directly and indirectly with microtubules and actin respectively. The later takes place by the interaction of CT-Cx43 with adaptor proteins such as zonula occludens-1 (ZO-1) and drebrin (developmentally regulated brain protein). Perturbation of this interaction has been implicated for the development of various developmental and cardiac defects (**Figure 3**) [87].

The growth suppressing effect of Cx43 was not compromised while expressing only CT-Cx-43 in HeLa cells [89] and HEK-293 cells [89]. CT-Cx-43 has been shown to have nuclear localization implying that it may be involved in regulating gene expression directly or indirectly within the nucleus [89]. In direct regulation it may act as a transcriptional activator or repressor of target genes however, in indirect regulation it may regulate target gene by acting as a transcriptional activator or repressor of miRNAs targeting them. In various cancers it has been shown the expression of one tumor suppressor gene can rescue the expression of other tumor suppressor gene as well [75, 90]. However the exact mechanism is not fully understood. P53 known to act as guardian of genome is a tumor suppressor playing very important role in regulating cellular process [91] such as cell proliferation [92, 93]. The expression of p53 increases under stress conditions [94] than its basal levels under normal condition [95]. These stress conditions include DNA damage [96] and oncogenic insults [97]. Dysregulation of p53 is considered to be initiator of tumorigenesis which includes its down regulation or mutation [98–100]. Expression of p53 has been found to be upregulated by CT-Cx43 in cardiomyocytes [88]. In addition, a group of small RNAs, i.e., microRNAs (miRNAs), has been shown to be able to regulate the expression of genes implicated in various normal and pathological conditions, including cellular proliferation and cancer [101–106]. More precisely a conserved homolog of *C. elegans* miRNA lin-4 namely miR-125b has been found to be dysregulated in various cancers [107]. The expressional studies of miR-125b in various cancers have revealed that miR-125b is upregulated in some cancers and

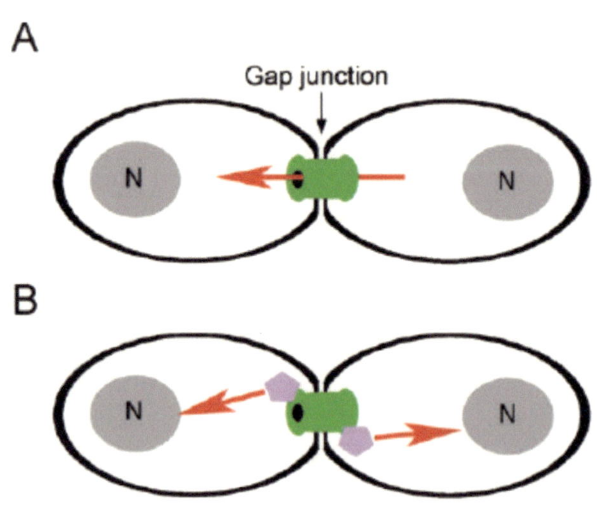

Figure 3.
Channel dependent and independent mechanisms by which Connexin expression can alter other genes. (A) Channel dependent mechanism. In this model, signaling molecules (red arrow) are directly exchanged between cell cytoplasms there by coordinately regulating gene expression patterns in the nucleus (N) (B) connexin dependent but channel independent mechanism. In this model connexins that may or may not be at junction membrane either bind a molecule with transcriptional activity (purple trapezoid) or can cleave such a portion of carboxy terminus to signal to the nucleus In this model connexins that may or may not be at junction membrane either bind a molecule with transcriptional activity (purple trapezoid) or can cleave such a portion of carboxy terminus to signal to the nucleus. Adapted from (Kardami et al., 2007) [88].

downregulated in others such as breast cancer. Therefore, it has occasionally been labeled as a tumor suppressor. Most of the dysregulated miRNAs has been shown to target tumor suppressor genes such as PTEN, RB, Cx43 and p53 [108, 109].

9. Connexin 43 as theurapatic target

Connexins have a dynamic role in the metastatic process, involving multiple factors. Metastasis is preceded by a series of events -tumor cells leave the primary tumor, move too far off sites and some start secondary tumors. While dealing with therapeutic issues, this variety of roles of connexins and GJIC in tumor development requires special attention. The anti-tumor growth function of connexins and their observed loss in cancer has made it clear that a possible strategy to inhibit tumor growth could be provided by restoring connexins expression. The targets of anti-cancer therapeutics are enzymes that affect global gene expression including HDAC, a set of enzymes involved in chromatin remodeling. Upon generation and testing of many HDAC inhibitors (HDACi), it has been observed that the effects of these drugs (at least some part of them) are GJIC-dependent. When prostate cancer cells were treated with the HDACi Trichostatin A (TSA) restoration of both Cx43 expression and GJIC takes place [110]. Hyperphosphorylation and degradation of Cx43 was also countered via the modulation of MAP kinases and Src [111]. Proteins that are involved in tumor progression and metastasis can regulate Connexin expression at transcriptional level. Cx43 is transcriptionally upregulated by the Ras–Raf-MAPK pathway via the interaction of its promoter with a protein complex that contains both HSP90 and c-Myc [112]. Protein AML1-ETO fusion protein transcriptionally upregulated Cx43 expression resulting from the chromosomal translocation t(8;21) frequently associated with acute myeloid leukemia (AML) via the JNK signaling pathway. The JNK specific inhibitor SP600125 was shown to inhibit this effect [55]. Melanoma metastasis was promoted by the protease-activated receptor-1 (PAR-1) via transcriptional regulation of Cx43 [54, 113]. The importance of Connexin phosphorylation, especially Cx43, in the regulation of their levels and functions has been extensively investigated [114]. The stability and degradation of Connexin proteins are regulated by the lysosomal and proteasomal systems, in addition to phosphorylation [113]. The efficacy of drugs could be improved by the stabilization of the Cx43 protein. For example, while sensitizing cells to the pro-apoptotic effect of MG132, the rate of degradation was decreased by treatment with the proteasome inhibitor MG132 [115]. A major regulatory event in the life of Connexins is phosphorylation by the kinase Src. Phosphorylation by Src takes place either directly or via signaling intermediates such as PKC and MAPK which resuls in a disruption of GJIC [116]. This effect has been shown to lead to drug resistance [117]. In colon cancer cells that already express Cx43 mRNA, Cx43 expression and phosphorylation were enhanced by Kaempferol, a plant flavonoid, via a Stat3-dependent mechanism. However, Kaempferol showed no effect in cells that were devoid of Cx43 mRNA and deficient in GJIC [118]. Therefore, targeting the post-translational modification of connexins is limited by the requirement of a functional transcriptional regulation. Such an isolated treatment would not be useful unless in combination with other treatments such as methylation- or acetylation-modulatory agents in order to unblock the transcription of c bvonnexins. In ovarian cancer cells, Cx43 phosphorylation and inhibition of GJIC was brought about by their treatment with endothelin-1 (ET-1), a ligand for the ETA receptor (ETAR), which is overexpressed in ovarian carcinoma [119]. The selective ETAR antagonist BQ 123, the tyrosine kinase inhibitor tyrphostin 25 or the c-Src inhibitor 4-amino-5-(4-chlorophenyl)-7-(t-butyl) pyrazolo [3, 4-d] pyramidine (PP2) blocked this effect, which suggests a role for Src in this mechanism [119]. Further, inhibition of ovarian tumor growth in vivo alongside a reduction of Cx43 phosphorylation was caused by ABT-627, an ETAR antagonist [119]. Summarily, the efficacy or specificity of these drugs can be increased by a combinatory approach considering an effect on both the Connexins and their regulatory molecules. In conclusion, gap junctional intercellular communication mediated by Connexins offer immense therapeutic opportunities that are still widely open. This approach is supported by original tools in the form of new findings regarding the regulation of Connexins expression. In view of the vast array of data about Connexins generated in various different tumor models and contexts, it is perhaps the right time for a consensus meeting devoted to focusing attention of the possibilities for Connexins as therapeutic targets.

Author details

Rabiya Rashid[1*], Shazia Ali[2*] and Mahboob-Ul-Hussain[1*]

1 Department of Biotechnology, University of Kashmir, India

2 CSIR IIIM, Srinagar, India

*Address all correspondence to: w.shazia@gmail.com, mahboob@uok.edu.in and rashid.rabiya@gmail.com

References

[1] Jensen HM. Preneoplastic lesions in the human breast. Science. 1976;191(4224):295-7.

[2] Razi S, Enayatrad M, Mohammadian-Hafshejani A, Salehiniya H. The epidemiology of skin cancer and its trend in Iran. International journal of preventive medicine. 2015;6:64.

[3] Zahedi A, Rafiemanesh H, Enayatrad M, Ghoncheh M, Salehiniya H. Incidence, trends and epidemiology of cancers in north west of Iran. Asian Pacific Journal of Cancer Prevention. 2015;16(16):7189-93.

[4] Ferlay J, Soerjomataram I, Dikshit R, Eser S, Mathers C, Rebelo M, et al. Cancer incidence and mortality worldwide: sources, methods and major patterns in GLOBOCAN 2012. International journal of cancer. 2015;136(5):E359-86.

[5] Clegg LX, Reichman ME, Miller BA, Hankey BF, Singh GK, Lin YD, et al. Impact of socioeconomic status on cancer incidence and stage at diagnosis: selected findings from the surveillance, epidemiology, and end results: National Longitudinal Mortality Study. Cancer causes & control. 2009;20(4):417-35.

[6] WHO | Breast cancer: prevention and control [Internet]. WHO. World Health Organization; [cited 2021 Jun 8]. Available from: http://www.who.int/cancer/detection/breastcancer/en/

[7] Youlden DR, Cramb SM, Yip CH, Baade PD. Incidence and mortality of female breast cancer in the Asia-Pacific region. Cancer biology & medicine. 2014;11(2):101-15.

[8] Choi Y, Kim Y, Park SK, Shin H-R, Yoo K-Y. Age-period-cohort analysis of female breast cancer mortality in Korea. Breast Cancer. 2006;13(3):266-71.

[9] Hoerger TJ, Ekwueme DU, Miller JW, Uzunangelov V, Hall IJ, Segel J, et al. Estimated effects of the national breast and cervical cancer early detection program on breast cancer mortality. American journal of preventive medicine. 2011;40(4):397-404.

[10] Ghoncheh M, Mohammadian-Hafshejani A, Salehiniya H. Incidence and mortality of breast cancer and their relationship to development in Asia. Asian Pacific Journal of Cancer Prevention. 2015;16(14):6081-7.

[11] Osuntokun BO. The changing pattern of disease in developing countries. In: World health forum 1985; 6 (4): 310-313. 1985.

[12] Wani MA, Jan FA, Khan NA, Pandita KK, Khurshid R, Khan SH. Cancer trends in Kashmir; common types, site incidence and demographic profiles: National Cancer Registry 2000-2012. Indian journal of cancer. 2014;51(2):133-7.

[13] Monaghan P, Clarke C, Perusinghe NP, Moss DW, Chen X-Y, Evans WH. Gap junction distribution and connexin expression in human breast. Experimental cell research. 1996;223(1):29-38.

[14] Chang C-C, Sun W, Cruz A, Saitoh M, Tai M-H, Trosko JE. A human breast epithelial cell type with stem cell characteristics as target cells for carcinogenesis. Radiation research. 2001;155(1):201-7.

[15] Nomata K, Kang K-S, Hayashi T, Matesic D, Lockwood L, Chang CC, et al. Inhibition of gap junctional intercellular communication in heptachlor-and heptachlor epoxide-treated normal human breast epithelial cells. Cell biology and toxicology. 1996;12(2):69-78.

[16] Trosko JE, Chang C-C, Wilson MR, Upham B, Hayashi T, Wade M. Gap junctions and the regulation of cellular functions of stem cells during development and differentiation. Methods. 2000;20(2):245-64.

[17] Lee SW, Tomasetto C, Paul D, Keyomarsi K, Sager R. Transcriptional downregulation of gap-junction proteins blocks junctional communication in human mammary tumor cell lines. The Journal of cell biology. 1992;118(5):1213-21.

[18] Hirschi KK, Xu CE, Tsukamoto T, Sager R. Gap junction genes Cx26 and Cx43 individually suppress the cancer phenotype of human mammary carcinoma cells and restore differentiation potential. Cell Growth and Differentiation-Publication American Association for Cancer Research. 1996;7(7):861-70.

[19] Laird DW, Fistouris P, Batist G, Alpert L, Huynh HT, Carystinos GD, et al. Deficiency of connexin43 gap junctions is an independent marker for breast tumors. Cancer research. 1999;59(16):4104-10.

[20] Li Z, Zhou Z, Welch DR, Donahue HJ. Expressing connexin 43 in breast cancer cells reduces their metastasis to lungs. Clinical & experimental metastasis. 2008;25(8):893-901.

[21] Naus CC, Elisevich K, Zhu D, Belliveau DJ, Del Maestro RF. In vivo growth of C6 glioma cells transfected with connexin43 cDNA. Cancer research. 1992;52(15):4208-13.

[22] Qin H, Shao Q, Curtis H, Galipeau J, Belliveau DJ, Wang T, et al. Retroviral delivery of connexin genes to human breast tumor cells inhibits in vivo tumor growth by a mechanism that is independent of significant gap junctional intercellular communication. Journal of Biological Chemistry. 2002;277(32):29132-8.

[23] Conklin CM, Bechberger JF, MacFabe D, Guthrie N, Kurowska EM, Naus CC. Genistein and quercetin increase connexin43 and suppress growth of breast cancer cells. Carcinogenesis. 2007;28(1):93-100.

[24] McLachlan E, Shao Q, Wang H, Langlois S, Laird DW. Connexins act as tumor suppressors in three-dimensional mammary cell organoids by regulating differentiation and angiogenesis. Cancer research. 2006;66(20):9886-94.

[25] Cairns RA, Khokha R, Hill RP. Molecular mechanisms of tumor invasion and metastasis: an integrated view. Current molecular medicine. 2003;3(7):659-71.

[26] Saunders MM, Seraj MJ, Li Z, Zhou Z, Winter CR, Welch DR, et al. Breast cancer metastatic potential correlates with a breakdown in homospecific and heterospecific gap junctional intercellular communication. Cancer research. 2001;61(5):1765-7.

[27] Momiyama M, Omori Y, Ishizaki Y, Nishikawa Y, Tokairin T, Ogawa J, et al. Connexin26-mediated gap junctional communication reverses the malignant phenotype of MCF-7 breast cancer cells. Cancer science. 2003;94(6):501-7.

[28] Kalra J, Shao Q, Qin H, Thomas T, Alaoui-Jamali MA, Laird DW. Cx26 inhibits breast MDA-MB-435 cell tumorigenic properties by a gap junctional intercellular communication-independent mechanism. Carcinogenesis. 2006;27(12):2528-37.

[29] Zhou D-R, Zhou Y-C, Cui G-H, Guo X, Qin J, Gui Y-T, et al. Gossypol repressed the gap junctional intercellular communication between Sertoli cells by decreasing the expression of Connexin43. Toxicology in vitro. 2008;22(7):1719-25.

[30] Cai J, Jiang WG, Mansel RE. Gap junctional communication and the

tyrosine phosphorylation of connexin 43 in interaction between breast cancer and endothelial cells. International journal of molecular medicine. 1998;1(1):273-81.

[31] Pollmann M-A, Shao Q, Laird DW, Sandig M. Connexin 43 mediated gap junctional communication enhances breast tumor cell diapedesis in culture. Breast Cancer Research. 2005;7(4):1-13.

[32] Mercer RR, Mastro AM. Cytokines secreted by bone-metastatic breast cancer cells alter the expression pattern of f-actin and reduce focal adhesion plaques in osteoblasts through PI3K. Experimental cell research. 2005;310(2):270-81.

[33] Mercer RR, Miyasaka C, Mastro AM. Metastatic breast cancer cells suppress osteoblast adhesion and differentiation. Clinical & experimental metastasis. 2004;21(5):427-35.

[34] Li Z, Zhou Z, Donahue HJ. Alterations in Cx43 and OB-cadherin affect breast cancer cell metastatic potential. Clinical & experimental metastasis. 2008;25(3):265-72.

[35] Hazan RB, Phillips GR, Qiao RF, Norton L, Aaronson SA. Exogenous expression of N-cadherin in breast cancer cells induces cell migration, invasion, and metastasis. The Journal of cell biology. 2000;148(4):779-90.

[36] Nieman MT, Prudoff RS, Johnson KR, Wheelock MJ. N-cadherin promotes motility in human breast cancer cells regardless of their E-cadherin expression. The Journal of cell biology. 1999;147(3):631-44.

[37] Huang R, Liu Y-G, Lin Y, Fan Y, Boynton A, Yang D, et al. Enhanced apoptosis under low serum conditions in human glioblastoma cells by connexin 43 (Cx43). Molecular Carcinogenesis: Published in cooperation with the University of Texas MD Anderson Cancer Center. 2001;32(3):128-38.

[38] Kanczuga-Koda L, Sulkowski S, Tomaszewski J, Koda M, Sulkowska M, Przystupa W, et al. Connexins 26 and 43 correlate with Bak, but not with Bcl-2 protein in breast cancer. Oncology reports. 2005;14(2):325-9.

[39] Vinken M, De Rop E, Decrock E, De Vuyst E, Leybaert L, Vanhaecke T, et al. Epigenetic regulation of gap junctional intercellular communication: more than a way to keep cells quiet? Biochimica et Biophysica Acta (BBA)-Reviews on Cancer. 2009;1795(1):53-61.

[40] Chen J-T, Cheng Y-W, Chou M-C, Sen-Lin T, Lai W-W, Ho WL, et al. The correlation between aberrant connexin 43 mRNA expression induced by promoter methylation and nodal micrometastasis in non-small cell lung cancer. Clinical Cancer Research. 2003;9(11):4200-4.

[41] Shimizu K, Onishi M, Sugata E, Sokuza Y, Mori C, Nishikawa T, et al. Disturbance of DNA methylation patterns in the early phase of hepatocarcinogenesis induced by a choline-deficient L-amino acid-defined diet in rats. Cancer science. 2007;98(9):1318-22.

[42] Tan L, Bianco T, Dobrovic A. Variable promoter region CpG island methylation of the putative tumor suppressor gene Connexin 26 in breast cancer. Carcinogenesis. 2002;23(2):231-6.

[43] Piechocki MP, Burk RD, Ruch RJ. Regulation of connexin32 and connexin43 gene expression by DNA methylation in rat liver cells. Carcinogenesis. 1999;20(3):401-6.

[44] DeSantis C, Ma J, Bryan L, Jemal A. Breast cancer statistics, 2013. CA: a cancer journal for clinicians. 2014;64(1):52-62.

[45] Parkin DM, Bray F, Ferlay J, Pisani P. Global cancer statistics, 2002. CA: a

cancer journal for clinicians. 2005;55(2):74-108.

[46] Coughlin SS, Ekwueme DU. Breast cancer as a global health concern. Cancer epidemiology. 2009;33(5):315-8.

[47] Jemal A, Center MM, DeSantis C, Ward EM. Global patterns of cancer incidence and mortality rates and trends. Cancer Epidemiology and Prevention Biomarkers. 2010;19(8):1893-907.

[48] Defamie N, Chepied A, Mesnil M. Connexins, gap junctions and tissue invasion. FEBS letters. 2014;588(8):1331-8.

[49] McLachlan E, Shao Q, Laird DW. Connexins and gap junctions in mammary gland development and breast cancer progression. Journal of Membrane Biology. 2007;218(1):107-21.

[50] Smyth JW, Shaw RM. Autoregulation of connexin43 gap junction formation by internally translated isoforms. Cell reports. 2013;5(3):611-8.

[51] Vliagoftis H, Ebeling C, Ilarraza R, Mahmudi-Azer S, Abel M, Adamko D, et al. Connexin 43 expression on peripheral blood eosinophils: role of gap junctions in transendothelial migration. BioMed research international. 2014;2014.

[52] Ryszawy D, Sarna M, Rak M, Szpak K, Kędracka-Krok S, Michalik M, et al. Functional links between Snail-1 and Cx43 account for the recruitment of Cx43-positive cells into the invasive front of prostate cancer. Carcinogenesis. 2014;35(9):1920-30.

[53] Fu Y, Jiang BQ, Wu Y, Li ZD, Zhuang ZG. Hsa-miR-206 inhibits the migration and invasion of breast cancer by targeting Cx43. Zhonghua yi xue za zhi. 2013;93(36):2890-4.

[54] Villares GJ, Dobroff AS, Wang H, Zigler M, Melnikova VO, Huang L, et al. Overexpression of protease-activated receptor-1 contributes to melanoma metastasis via regulation of connexin 43. Cancer research. 2009;69(16):6730-7.

[55] Gao F-H, Wang Q, Wu Y-L, Li XI, Zhao K-W, Chen G-Q. c-Jun N-terminal kinase mediates AML1-ETO protein-induced connexin-43 expression. Biochemical and biophysical research communications. 2007;356(2):505-11.

[56] Ming J, Zhou Y, Du J, Fan S, Pan B, Wang Y, et al. Identification of miR-200a as a novel suppressor of connexin 43 in breast cancer cells. Bioscience reports. 2015;35(5).

[57] Schmidt K, de Wit C. Keep calm and carry on: miR-1298 prevents up-regulation of Cx43 and secures a quiescent vascular smooth muscle cell. Cardiovasc Res. 2015;107:407-9.

[58] Fellmann C, Hoffmann T, Sridhar V, Hopfgartner B, Muhar M, Roth M, et al. An optimized microRNA backbone for effective single-copy RNAi. Cell reports. 2013;5(6):1704-13.

[59] Ghosh T, Aprea J, Nardelli J, Engel H, Selinger C, Mombereau C, et al. MicroRNAs establish robustness and adaptability of a critical gene network to regulate progenitor fate decisions during cortical neurogenesis. Cell reports. 2014;7(6):1779-88.

[60] Pollock A, Bian S, Zhang C, Chen Z, Sun T. Growth of the developing cerebral cortex is controlled by microRNA-7 through the p53 pathway. Cell reports. 2014;7(4):1184-96.

[61] Benaich N, Woodhouse S, Goldie SJ, Mishra A, Quist SR, Watt FM. Rewiring of an epithelial differentiation factor, miR-203, to inhibit human squamous cell carcinoma metastasis. Cell reports. 2014;9(1):104-17.

[62] Schober A, Nazari-Jahantigh M, Weber C. MicroRNA-mediated mechanisms of the cellular stress response in atherosclerosis. Nature Reviews Cardiology. 2015;12(6):361.

[63] Anderson C, Catoe H, Werner R. MIR-206 regulates connexin43 expression during skeletal muscle development. Nucleic acids research. 2006;34(20):5863-71.

[64] Yang B, Lin H, Xiao J, Lu Y, Luo X, Li B, et al. The muscle-specific microRNA miR-1 regulates cardiac arrhythmogenic potential by targeting GJA1 and KCNJ2. Nature medicine. 2007;13(4):486-91.

[65] Kanter HL, Saffitz JE, Beyer EC. Cardiac myocytes express multiple gap junction proteins. Circulation research. 1992;70(2):438-44.

[66] Ou C-W, Orsino A, Lye SJ. Expression of connexin-43 and connexin-26 in the rat myometrium during pregnancy and labor is differentially regulated by mechanical and hormonal signals. Endocrinology. 1997;138(12):5398-407.

[67] Lang LM, Beyer EC, Schwartz AL, Gitlin JD. Molecular cloning of a rat uterine gap junction protein and analysis of gene expression during gestation. American Journal of Physiology-Endocrinology And Metabolism. 1991;260(5):E787-93.

[68] Lefebvre DL, Piersanti M, Bai X-H, Chen Z-Q, Lye SJ. Myometrial transcriptional regulation of the gap junction gene, connexin-43. Reproduction, Fertility and Development. 1995;7(3):603-11.

[69] Piersanti M, Lye SJ. Increase in messenger ribonucleic acid encoding the myometrial gap junction protein, connexin-43, requires protein synthesis and is associated with increased expression of the activator protein-1, c-fos. Endocrinology. 1995;136(8):3571-8.

[70] Yu W, Dahl G, Werner R. The connexin43 gene is responsive to oestrogen. Proceedings of the Royal Society of London Series B: Biological Sciences. 1994;255(1343):125-32.

[71] Maroto FG, Sierra JM. Translational control in heat-shocked Drosophila embryos. Evidence for the inactivation of initiation factor (s) involved in the recognition of mRNA cap structure. Journal of Biological Chemistry. 1988;263(30):15720-5.

[72] Stein I, Itin A, Einat P, Skaliter R, Grossman Z, Keshet E. Translation of vascular endothelial growth factor mRNA by internal ribosome entry: implications for translation under hypoxia. Molecular and cellular biology. 1998;18(6):3112-9.

[73] Morris JA, Dorner AJ, Edwards CA, Hendershot LM, Kaufman RJ. Immunoglobulin binding protein (BiP) function is required to protect cells from endoplasmic reticulum stress but is not required for the secretion of selective proteins. Journal of Biological Chemistry. 1997;272(7):4327-34.

[74] Yanagisawa-Miwa A, Uchida Y, Nakamura F, Tomaru T, Kido H, Kamijo T, et al. Salvage of infarcted myocardium by angiogenic action of basic fibroblast growth factor. Science. 1992;257(5075):1401-3.

[75] Smith SI, Weil D, Johnson GR, Boyd AW, Li CL. Expression of the Wilms' tumor suppressor gene, WT1, is upregulated by leukemia inhibitory factor and induces monocytic differentiation in M1 leukemic cells. Blood, The Journal of the American Society of Hematology. 1998;91(3):764-73.

[76] Kanno Y, Loewenstein WR. Intercellular diffusion. Science. 1964;143(3609):959-60.

[77] Lawrence TS, Beers WH, Gilula NB. Transmission of hormonal stimulation by cell-to-cell communication. Nature. 1978;272(5653):501-6.

[78] Willecke K, Eiberger J, Degen J, Eckardt D, Romualdi A, Güldenagel M, et al. Structural and functional diversity of connexin genes in the mouse and human genome. Biological chemistry. 2002;383(5):725-37.

[79] Pointis G, Gilleron J, Carette D, Segretain D. Physiological and physiopathological aspects of connexins and communicating gap junctions in spermatogenesis. Philosophical Transactions of the Royal Society B: Biological Sciences. 2010;365(1546):1607-20.

[80] Sirnes S, Bruun J, Kolberg M, Kjenseth A, Lind GE, Svindland A, et al. Connexin43 acts as a colorectal cancer tumor suppressor and predicts disease outcome. International journal of cancer. 2012;131(3):570-81.

[81] Ismail R, Rashid R, Andrabi K, Parray FQ, Besina S, Shah MA, et al. Pathological implications of Cx43 down-regulation in human colon cancer. Asian Pacific Journal of Cancer Prevention. 2014;15(7):2987-91.

[82] Oyamada M, Oyamada Y, Takamatsu T. Regulation of connexin expression. Biochimica et Biophysica Acta (BBA)-Biomembranes. 2005;1719(1-2):6-23.

[83] Moorby C, Patel M. Dual functions for connexins: Cx43 regulates growth independently of gap junction formation. Experimental cell research. 2001;271(2):238-48.

[84] King TJ, Bertram JS. Connexins as targets for cancer chemoprevention and chemotherapy. Biochimica et Biophysica Acta (BBA)-Biomembranes. 2005;1719(1-2):146-60.

[85] Trosko JE, Ruch RJ. Gap junctions as targets for cancer chemoprevention and chemotherapy. Current Drug Targets. 2002;3(6):465-82.

[86] Retamal MA, Cortés CJ, Reuss L, Bennett MV, Sáez JC. S-nitrosylation and permeation through connexin 43 hemichannels in astrocytes: induction by oxidant stress and reversal by reducing agents. Proceedings of the National Academy of Sciences. 2006;103(12):4475-80.

[87] Leithe E, Mesnil M, Aasen T. The connexin 43 C-terminus: A tail of many tales. Biochimica et Biophysica Acta (BBA)-Biomembranes. 2018;1860(1):48-64.

[88] Kardami E, Dang X, Iacobas DA, Nickel BE, Jeyaraman M, Srisakuldee W, et al. The role of connexins in controlling cell growth and gene expression. Progress in biophysics and molecular biology. 2007;94(1-2):245-64.

[89] Dang X, Doble BW, Kardami E. The carboxy-tail of connexin-43 localizes to the nucleus and inhibits cell growth. Molecular and cellular biochemistry. 2003;242(1):35-8.

[90] Hsu T-H, Chu C-C, Jiang S-Y, Hung M-W, Ni W-C, Lin H-E, et al. Expression of the class II tumor suppressor gene RIG1 is directly regulated by p53 tumor suppressor in cancer cell lines. FEBS letters. 2012;586(9):1287-93.

[91] Foulkes WD. p53–master and commander. N engl j med. 2007;357(25):2539-41.

[92] Sulzyc-Bielicka V, Domagala P, Bielicki D, Safranow K, Domagala W. Thymidylate synthase expression and p21 WAF1/p53 phenotype of colon cancers identify patients who may benefit from 5-fluorouracil based therapy. Cellular Oncology. 2014;37(1):17-28.

[93] Wawryk-Gawda E, Chylińska-Wrzos P, Lis-Sochocka M, Chłapek K, Bulak K, Jędrych M, et al. P53 protein in proliferation, repair and apoptosis of cells. Protoplasma. 2014;251(3):525-33.

[94] Giaccia AJ, Kastan MB. The complexity of p53 modulation: emerging patterns from divergent signals. Genes & development. 1998;12(19):2973-83.

[95] Almog N, Rotter V. Involvement of p53 in cell differentiation and development. Biochimica et biophysica acta. 1997;1333(1):F1-27.

[96] Sakaguchi K, Herrera JE, Saito S, Miki T, Bustin M, Vassilev A, et al. DNA damage activates p53 through a phosphorylation–acetylation cascade. Genes & development. 1998;12(18):2831-41.

[97] Lowe SW. Activation of p53 by oncogenes. Endocrine-related cancer. 1999;6(1):45-8.

[98] Muller PA, Vousden KH. p53 mutations in cancer. Nature cell biology. 2013;15(1):2-8.

[99] Rivlin N, Brosh R, Oren M, Rotter V. Mutations in the p53 tumor suppressor gene: important milestones at the various steps of tumorigenesis. Genes & cancer. 2011;2(4):466-74.

[100] Zheng L, Ren JQ, Hua LI, Kong ZL, Zhu HG. Downregulation of wild-type p53 protein by HER-2/neu mediated PI3K pathway activation in human breast cancer cells: its effect on cell proliferation and implication for therapy. Cell research. 2004;14(6):497-506.

[101] Maqbool R, Hussain MU. MicroRNAs and human diseases: diagnostic and therapeutic potential. Cell and tissue research. 2014;358(1):1-15.

[102] Nagadia R, Pandit P, Coman WB, Cooper-White J, Punyadeera C. miRNAs in head and neck cancer revisited. Cellular Oncology. 2013;36(1):1-7.

[103] Rask L, Balslev E, Søkilde R, Høgdall E, Flyger H, Eriksen J, et al. Differential expression of miR-139, miR-486 and miR-21 in breast cancer patients sub-classified according to lymph node status. Cellular Oncology. 2014;37(3):215-27.

[104] Salazar C, Nagadia R, Pandit P, Cooper-White J, Banerjee N, Dimitrova N, et al. A novel saliva-based microRNA biomarker panel to detect head and neck cancers. Cellular Oncology. 2014;37(5):331-8.

[105] Hussain MU. Micro-RNAs (miRNAs): genomic organisation, biogenesis and mode of action. Cell and tissue research. 2012;349(2):405-13.

[106] Wang Y, Li M, Zang W, Ma Y, Wang N, Li P, et al. MiR-429 up-regulation induces apoptosis and suppresses invasion by targeting Bcl-2 and SP-1 in esophageal carcinoma. Cellular oncology. 2013;36(5):385-94.

[107] Banzhaf-Strathmann J, Edbauer D. Good guy or bad guy: the opposing roles of microRNA 125b in cancer. Cell communication and signaling. 2014;12(1):1-13.

[108] Tsang WP, Ng EK, Ng SS, Jin H, Yu J, Sung JJ, et al. Oncofetal H19-derived miR-675 regulates tumor suppressor RB in human colorectal cancer. Carcinogenesis. 2010;31(3):350-8.

[109] Zhu S, Wu H, Wu F, Nie D, Sheng S, Mo Y-Y. MicroRNA-21 targets tumor suppressor genes in invasion and metastasis. Cell research. 2008;18(3):350-9.

[110] Hernandez M, Shao Q, Yang X-J, Luh S-P, Kandouz M, Batist G, et al. A

histone deacetylation-dependent mechanism for transcriptional repression of the gap junction gene cx43 in prostate cancer cells. The Prostate. 2006;66(11):1151-61.

[111] Jung J-W, Cho S-D, Ahn N-S, Yang S-R, Park J-S, Jo E-H, et al. Effects of the histone deacetylases inhibitors sodium butyrate and trichostatin A on the inhibition of gap junctional intercellular communication by H2O2-and 12-O-tetradecanoylphorbol-13-acetate in rat liver epithelial cells. Cancer letters. 2006;241(2):301-8.

[112] Carystinos GD, Kandouz M, Alaoui-Jamali MA, Batist G. Unexpected induction of the human connexin 43 promoter by the ras signaling pathway is mediated by a novel putative promoter sequence. Molecular pharmacology. 2003;63(4):821-31.

[113] Leithe E, Rivedal E. Ubiquitination of gap junction proteins. Journal of Membrane Biology. 2007;217(1):43-51.

[114] Solan JL, Lampe PD. Connexin43 phosphorylation: structural changes and biological effects. Biochemical Journal. 2009;419(2):261-72.

[115] Huang Q, Liu XZ, Kang CS, Wang GX, Zhong Y, Pu PY. The anti-glioma effect of suicide gene therapy using BMSC expressing HSV/TK combined with overexpression of Cx43 in glioma cells. Cancer gene therapy. 2010;17(3):192-202.

[116] Pahujaa M, Anikin M, Goldberg GS. Phosphorylation of connexin43 induced by Src: regulation of gap junctional communication between transformed cells. Experimental cell research. 2007;313(20):4083-90.

[117] Brissette JL, Kumar NM, Gilula NB, Dotto GP. The tumor promoter 12-O-tetradecanoylphorbol-13-acetate and the ras oncogene modulate expression and phosphorylation of gap junction proteins. Molecular and Cellular Biology. 1991;11(10):5364-71.

[118] Nakamura Y, Chang C-C, Mori T, Sato K, Ohtsuki K, Upham BL, et al. Augmentation of differentiation and gap junction function by kaempferol in partially differentiated colon cancer cells. Carcinogenesis. 2005;26(3):665-71.

[119] Spinella F, Rosanò L, Di Castro V, Nicotra MR, Natali PG, Bagnato A. Endothelin-1 decreases gap junctional intercellular communication by inducing phosphorylation of connexin 43 in human ovarian carcinoma cells. Journal of Biological Chemistry. 2003;278(42):41294-301.